BASIC LIFE SUPPORT AND AED FOR HEALTHCARE PRACTITIONERS

A STEP-BY-STEP GUIDE

Blessing Isaackson

Ebook ISBN: 978-1-7385061-0-1

Paperback ISBN: 978-1-7385061-3-2

Table of Contents

FOREWORD

Fairview Training is committed to providing high-quality learning resources that support learners to meet their continuing professional development (CPD) requirements.

This step-by-step guide has been written to help healthcare professionals consolidate their basic life support and AED skills. It is intended to complement face-to-face training and to serve as a reference during and after the course.

Blessing Isaackson

Managing Director

FAIRVIEW TRAINING LTD

Principles of Basic Life Support

Aims of providing basic life support.

Preserve life
Maintain circulation, airway, and breathing to keep the person alive until advanced care is available.

Prevent deterioration
Stop the condition from worsening by early recognition, prompt calling for help, and timely CPR and defibrillation.

Promote recovery
Improve survival and neurological outcome through high-quality CPR, early defibrillation, and safe ongoing care until handover.

AIMS OF PROVIDING BASIC LIFE SUPPORT

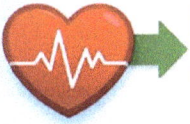

Preserve Life

Keep the patient alive.

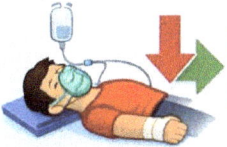

Prevent Deterioration

Stop the condition from worsening.

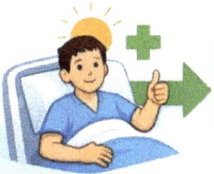

Promote Recovery

Help the patient heal.

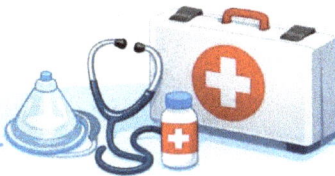

Minimising the Risk of Infection (PPE)

Infection prevention and control measures must be followed in line with **current healthcare guidance**, local policy, and dynamic risk assessment.

Healthcare practitioners should use **standard precautions for all patients** and additional measures where infection is suspected.

Appropriate PPE may include:

- Disposable **gloves**
- Disposable **apron or gown**
- **Surgical face mask** or **respirator (e.g. FFP3)** if aerosol-generating procedures are anticipated
- **Eye/face protection** (visor or face shield)

Hand hygiene must be performed before and after patient contact. PPE should be removed and disposed of safely. **Life-saving treatment should not be delayed** if PPE is not immediately available.

Alerting the emergency services

- **Call 999 (UK) or 112** as a matter of urgency.
- **In UK NHS hospitals, call 2222** and state the location clearly.
- If alone with a mobile phone, activate emergency services using speakerphone **as soon as cardiac arrest is suspected**, then commence CPR immediately. (Adult BLS emphasis: call first for any unresponsive person.) (Resuscitation Council UK)

Communication, SBAR & Consent

1. The Importance of Communication

Effective communication is fundamental to **safe, ethical, and high-quality healthcare**. Clear and professional communication:

- Protects patients from harm
- Builds trust, confidence, and therapeutic relationships
- Reduces errors, misunderstandings, and complaints
- Supports compliance with professional standards, ethical guidance, and legal requirements

Healthcare professionals communicate not only with patients, but also with **colleagues and external services**, including emergency services, specialist teams, hospitals, primary care providers, and other multidisciplinary professionals.

Communicating with Patients

Clear, Simple, and Accessible Communication

Healthcare professionals should ensure that information is communicated in a way patients can understand:

- Avoid unnecessary clinical jargon; explain conditions and procedures in plain language
- Break information into manageable sections
- Check understanding using open-ended questions (e.g. *"Can you explain in your own words what we have discussed?"*)

Patient-Centred Approach

- Listen actively and acknowledge patient concerns
- Tailor communication for patients with anxiety, cognitive impairment, learning disabilities, sensory impairment, or language barriers
- Use interpreters, advocates, or communication aids when required
- Communication should be **a two-way process**, encouraging patient involvement and shared decision-making

SBAR: A Structured Communication Tool

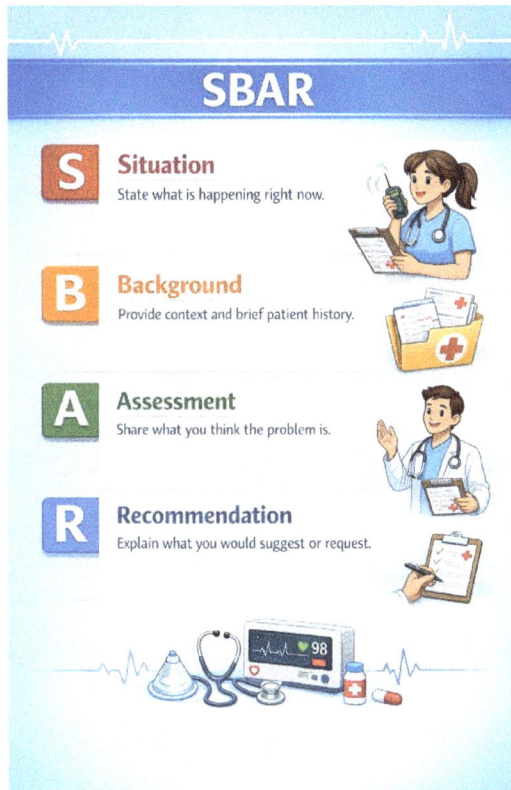

SBAR is a nationally recognised framework used to communicate clinical information **clearly, concisely, and safely**, particularly in urgent or high-risk situations.

Letter	Meaning	Purpose
S	Situation	What is happening now
B	Background	Relevant history or context
A	Assessment	What you think the problem is
R	Recommendation	What needs to happen next

Example: Medical Emergency

- **S:** "I am calling from a clinical setting. I have a patient with suspected anaphylaxis."
- **B:** "They were given medication and rapidly developed wheeze and hypotension."
- **A:** "They are conscious but in respiratory distress."
- **R:** "We need an emergency ambulance immediately."

SBAR is particularly useful for:

- Emergency service calls
- Clinical handovers
- Escalating concerns within healthcare teams
- Communicating across multidisciplinary teams

Understanding Consent

Consent is a patient's agreement to receive care or treatment. For consent to be valid, it must be:

- **Voluntary**

- **Informed**
- **Given by a person with capacity**

These principles are defined in professional standards and UK law.

Types of Consent

- **Implied:** Patient cooperation with routine care (e.g. presenting an arm for blood pressure measurement)
- **Verbal:** Most routine assessments and treatments
- **Written:** Complex, invasive, or high-risk procedures

What Makes Consent Valid?

1. Capacity

Under the **Mental Capacity Act 2005**, a patient has capacity if they can:

- Understand relevant information
- Retain the information
- Weigh the information to decide
- Communicate their decision

Adults are presumed to have capacity unless there is evidence to suggest otherwise.

2. Information

Patients must be given sufficient information about:

- The nature and purpose of the intervention
- Expected benefits and material risks
- Reasonable alternatives, including no treatment
- Potential consequences of declining treatment

3. Voluntariness

- Consent must be given freely, without pressure or coercion
- Patients have the right to refuse or withdraw consent at any time
- Consent is an **ongoing process**, not a one-off event

Special Consent Situations

Children and Young People

- Assess decision-making capacity (e.g. Gillick competence)
- If the child lacks capacity, consent must be obtained from a person with parental responsibility

Medical Emergencies

- If a patient lacks capacity and delay would result in serious harm or death, treatment may proceed in the patient's **best interests**
- The decision-making process and rationale must be clearly documented

7. Documentation

Accurate, timely, and clear records are essential and should include:

- Information provided to the patient
- Questions asked and responses given
- The type of consent obtained
- Any refusal or withdrawal of consent

Good documentation protects **both patients and healthcare professionals** and supports safe, accountable practice.

DNACPR (Do Not Attempt Cardiopulmonary Resuscitation)

A **DNACPR** is a formal clinical decision indicating that **cardiopulmonary resuscitation (CPR) should not be attempted** in the event of cardiac arrest.

- A DNACPR decision applies **only to CPR**
- It does **not** mean that other care should be withheld
- All appropriate treatment and supportive care must continue, including:
    - Oxygen therapy
    - Airway management
    - Pain relief
    - Symptom control and comfort measures

Respecting a DNACPR Decision

Honouring a DNACPR decision:

- Respects **patient autonomy** and previously expressed wishes
- Preserves **dignity and comfort** at the end of life
- Prevents **inappropriate or potentially harmful interventions**

Responsibilities of Healthcare Professionals

Healthcare professionals should:

- Be aware of existing DNACPR decisions when caring for patients
- Check and verify DNACPR documentation where possible
- Communicate clearly within the healthcare team
- Follow **national and local guidance** if there is uncertainty or disagreement

A DNACPR decision does **not** replace clinical judgement and should always be considered within the wider context of the patient's care plan.

PRIMARY SURVEY

PRIMARY SURVEY – DRS ABC

The **Primary Survey (DRS ABC)** is a structured, rapid assessment used to identify and manage **immediate life-threatening problems**.
Each step is completed **in order**, and any problems found are addressed **before moving on**.

D – Danger

Check for danger to yourself, the patient, and others.

- Look for hazards (e.g. traffic, sharps, electrical risks, body fluids, equipment)
- Use appropriate PPE where available
- Do **not** approach until the scene is safe

R – Response

Assess the patient's level of responsiveness.

- Speak loudly: *"Can you hear me?"*
- Gently shake the shoulders (adults and children)
- In infants: stimulate by tapping the soles of the feet

If responsive:

- Leave in the position found (if safe)
- Monitor closely and seek appropriate help

If unresponsive:

- Proceed immediately to **Shout for Help**

S – Shout for Help

Call for assistance early.

- Shout for help from nearby staff or bystanders
- Activate emergency response:
  - **999 or 112** (community)
  - **2222** in UK hospital settings
- If alone, use a mobile phone on speaker mode while continuing care

A – Airway

Open and assess the airway.

- Use **head tilt–chin lift**
- Look for visible obstruction (vomit, blood, foreign body)
- Remove visible obstructions **only if safe**
- If trauma suspected, follow local policy (e.g. jaw thrust)

An obstructed airway is **immediately life-threatening** and must be managed before proceeding.

B – Breathing

Assess breathing for no more than 10 seconds.

- Look for chest movement
- Listen for breath sounds
- Feel for airflow on your cheek

Normal breathing:

- Place in the recovery position if unresponsive
- Monitor continuously

Not breathing or abnormal breathing (agonal gasps):

- Treat as cardiac arrest
- Proceed immediately to **CPR**

C – CPR & Circulation

Start CPR if the patient is not breathing normally.

Chest Compressions (Adult)

- Centre of the chest
- Depth: **5–6 cm**
- Rate: **100–120 per minute**
- Allow full chest recoil
- Minimise interruptions

Compression–Ventilation Ratio

- **30 compressions : 2 breaths** (if trained and willing)
- If unable or unwilling to give breaths: **compression-only CPR**

Defibrillation

- Send for and use an **AED as soon as available**
- Follow voice prompts
- Resume CPR immediately after shock or if no shock advised

Key Clinical Points

- **DRS ABC is a continuous cycle** – reassess frequently
- Abnormal or absent breathing = **cardiac arrest**
- **Early CPR and early defibrillation save lives**
- If in doubt, **start chest compressions**

PRIMARY SURVEY
DRS ABC

D **Danger**
Check for hazards to
yourself and the casualty.

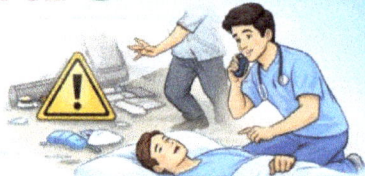

R **Response**
Assess responsiveness (talk & tap).

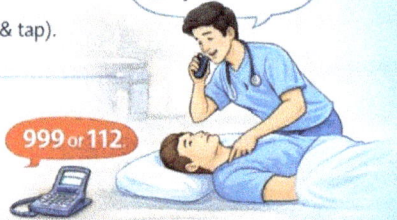

S **Shout for Help**
Alert emergency services
immediately.

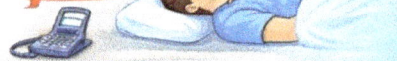

A **Airway**
Open the airway (head tilt–chin lift).

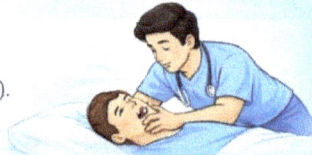

B **Breathing**
Look, listen, feel for up to 10 seconds.

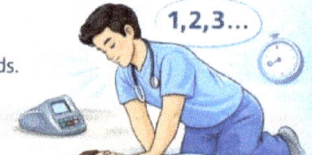

C **CPR & Circulation**
Start chest compressions
if not breathing normally.

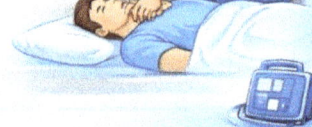

Chain of Survival

The **2025 Resuscitation Council UK chain of survival** highlights:

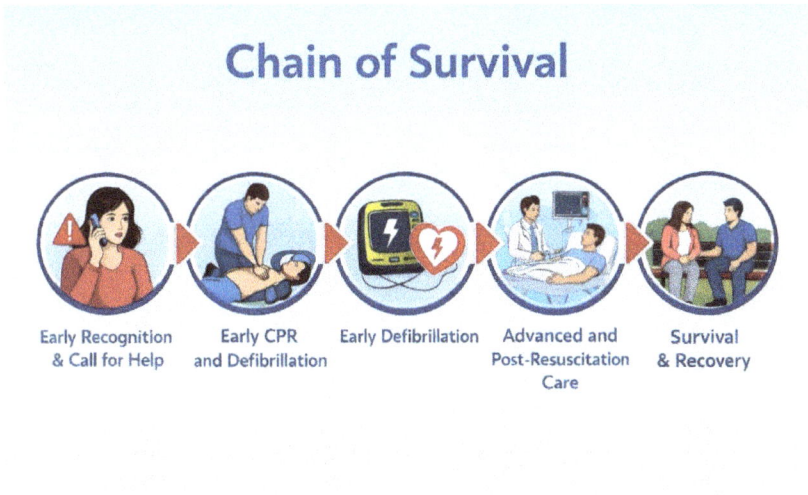

1. Early Recognition & Call for Help

Identify cardiac arrest quickly by checking responsiveness and breathing. Activate emergency services immediately so the right help is on the way.

2. Early CPR and Defibrillation

Start high-quality chest compressions without delay and use an AED as soon as it becomes available. These two actions together give the best chance of restoring a shockable rhythm.

3. Advanced and Post-Resuscitation Care

Once professionals arrive, they provide advanced life support, treat reversible causes, stabilise the patient, and deliver structured post-ROSC care in the hospital.

4. Survival & Recovery

Ongoing hospital treatment, rehabilitation, and psychological support help the patient recover and return to daily life.

Calling for Help

Call **999 or 112** immediately and provide clear, accurate information, including:

- **Your exact location**
- **The type of emergency and help required**
- **The patient's name** (if known)
- **The number of patients involved**

In an **NHS hospital environment in the UK**, activate the emergency response by calling **2222** and clearly stating the location and nature of the emergency.

Assessing Vital Signs

Assessment of vital signs should be performed as part of a **systematic clinical assessment**, such as **DRABCDE**, and repeated regularly to detect deterioration.[19]

Airway

- Ensure the airway is **open and patent**
- Look for visible obstruction (e.g. foreign body, vomit, swelling)
- Listen for abnormal sounds such as stridor or gurgling
- If compromised, **airway management takes immediate priority**

Breathing

- Assess **rate, depth, rhythm, and effort**
- Normal adult respiratory rate: **12–20 breaths per minute**
- Measure oxygen saturation using pulse oximetry where available:
  - **Target SpO$_2$: 94–98%** in most adults
  - **Target SpO$_2$: 88–92%** in patients at risk of hypercapnic respiratory failure (e.g. COPD), if known[20]
- Look for signs of respiratory distress (cyanosis, accessory muscle use)

Circulation

Assess perfusion and cardiovascular status:

- **Pulse**
  - Check **carotid** pulse in unresponsive adults
  - Radial or brachial pulse may be used in conscious patients
  - Note rate, rhythm, and strength
- **Blood pressure**
  - Normal adult BP is approximately **120/80 mmHg**

- - Interpret in context of symptoms and baseline
- **Capillary refill time**
  - Normal: **≤2 seconds** (in adults, measured centrally if shocked)
- Look for signs of shock: pallor, sweating, tachycardia, hypotension[21]

Temperature

- Normal adult body temperature: **36.0–37.5°C**
- **Hypothermia**
  - Mild: **32–35°C**
  - Moderate: **28–32°C**
  - Severe: **<28°C**
- **Hyperthermia**
  - **Heat exhaustion**: raised temperature with preserved consciousness
  - **Heat stroke: core temperature ≥40°C with altered mental status**
    → This is a **medical emergency**[22]

Key Clinical Points for Practice

- Always **call for help early** if concerned
- Vital signs must be interpreted **together**, not in isolation
- Abnormal findings require **prompt escalation and reassessment**
- Repeated observations help identify **deterioration**

References (continuing numbering)

18. NHS England. *Emergency Call Handling and Communication Guidance*

19.Resuscitation Council UK. *Primary Survey and Assessment of the Acutely Ill Adult*
20.British Thoracic Society. *Guideline for Oxygen Use in Adults in Healthcare and Emergency Settings*
21.NICE. *Acutely Ill Adults in Hospital: Recognition and Response to Deterioration*
22.UK Health Security Agency. *Heat Illness and Hyperthermia Guidance*

Temperature

Digital Thermometer

Digital thermometers are commonly used in clinical practice and can measure temperature via the **oral, axillary (armpit), or rectal** routes, depending on the device and patient factors. **Core temperature measurement methods** (such as rectal measurement) are the most accurate. **Oral, axillary, tympanic, and temporal measurements** may be less reliable and can be influenced by factors such as technique, patient condition, and environment.

The choice of measurement site should follow **local policy, clinical context, and patient suitability**.

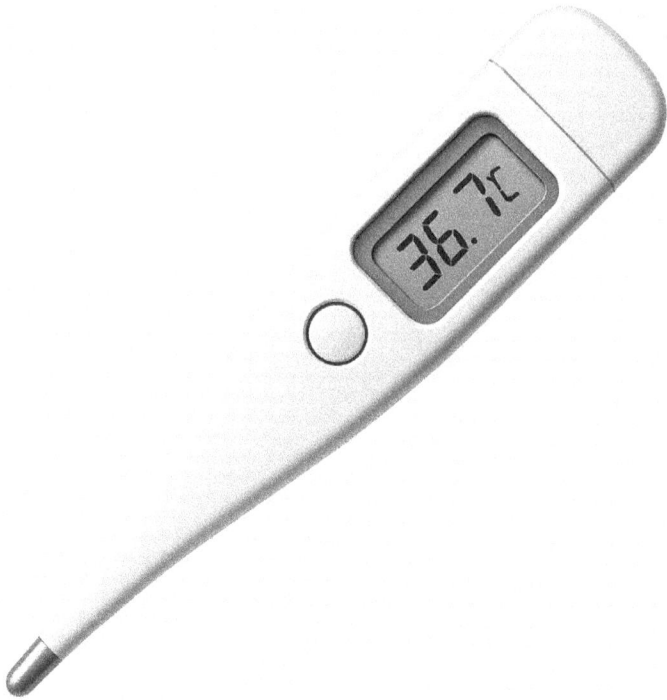

Tympanic Thermometer: is a thermometer that measures the temperature inside the patient's ears by measuring the infrared heat inside the ear.

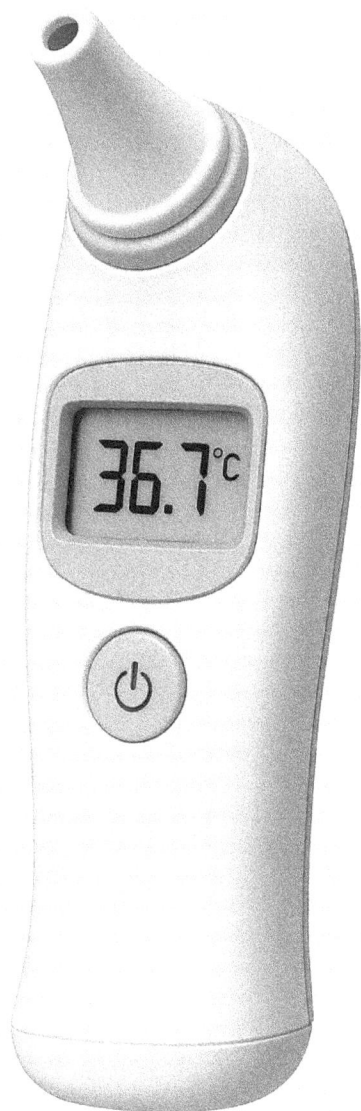

Temporal Thermometer-forehead thermometer. They are not as dependable as digital thermometers. They are placed or pointed at the forehead. They measure the infrared heat generated by the forehead.

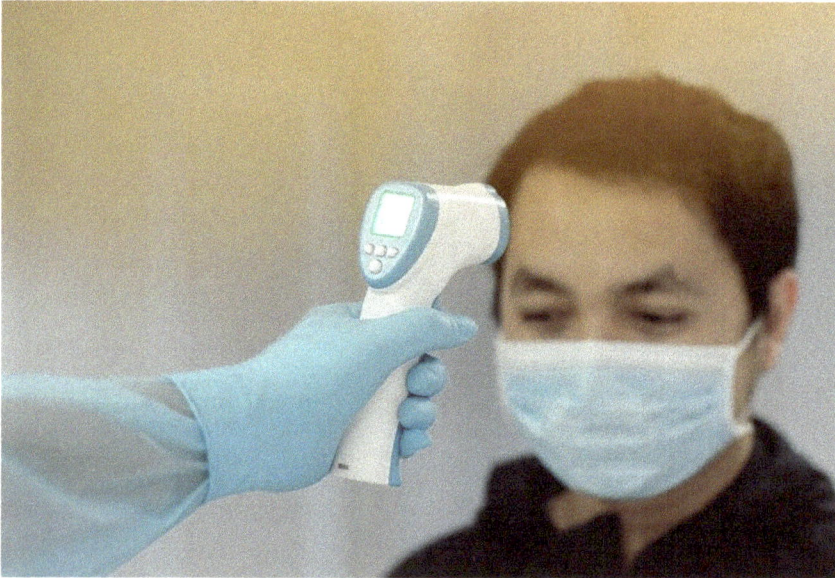

Pulse

The pulse is the detectable pressure wave created when the heart contracts and blood moves through the arteries. It is used to determine heart rate, typically measured in beats per minute (bpm), and to assess the rhythm, strength, and regularity of heart function.

In basic life support, cardiac arrest is identified by unresponsiveness and the absence of normal breathing. Healthcare professionals trained in pulse checking may assess for a pulse for no more than 10 seconds. If there is any doubt, commence chest compressions."

Pulse Locations (Adult)

Peripheral and central pulse assessment is a vital part of clinical evaluation, especially in emergency situations. The choice of pulse site depends on the patient's age, level of consciousness, and overall clinical condition.

Common Pulse Sites

Carotid Pulse (Central)

- Found on either side of the neck, in the space between the trachea and the sternocleidomastoid muscle
- Only one side should be assessed at a time to prevent reduced blood flow to the brain
- Serves as the primary pulse site for evaluating unresponsive adults[23]

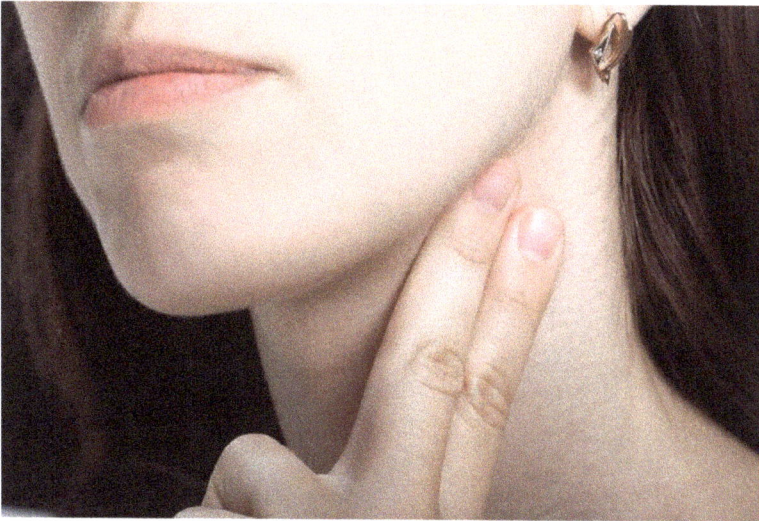

Brachial Pulse (Peripheral)

- Located on the inner side of the upper arm, between the biceps and triceps muscles
- Commonly assessed in infants and children, but may also be used in adults when other pulse sites are difficult to detect[24]

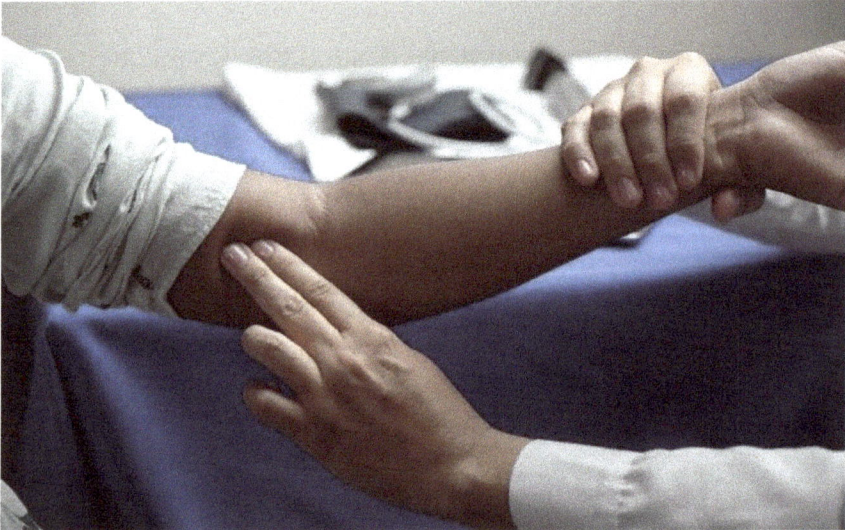

Femoral Pulse (Central)

- Located in the upper thigh, just below the inguinal ligament, midway between the anterior superior iliac spine and the pubic symphysis
- Particularly useful in cases of shock, cardiac arrest, or other low-flow states[23]

Radial Pulse (Peripheral)

- Located on the thumb side of the wrist, between the radius and the flexor tendons
- Commonly assessed in conscious adults to evaluate pulse rate and rhythm

Let me know if you would like all pulse descriptions formatted uniformly for a study guide or manual.

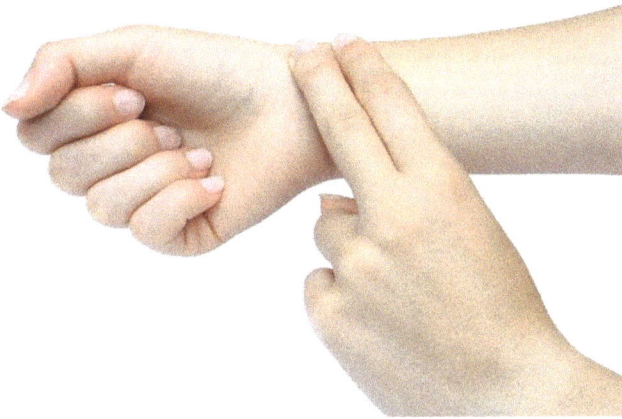

Popliteal Pulse (Peripheral)

· Located behind the knee in the popliteal fossa

· Often difficult to palpate and requires the knee to ᵇ slightly flexed

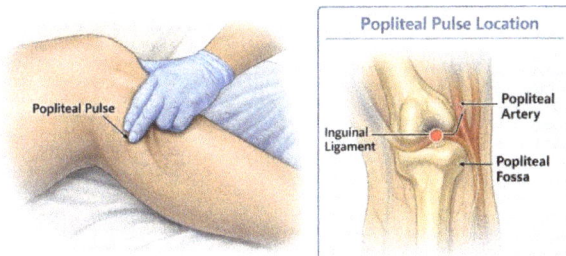

Popliteal Pulse

Popliteal Pulse Location

Popliteal Artery

Inguinal Ligament

Popliteal Fossa

Posterior Tibial Pulse (Peripheral)

- Located posterior to and slightly below the medial malleolus (inner ankle bone)
- Used to assess peripheral circulation in the lower limb

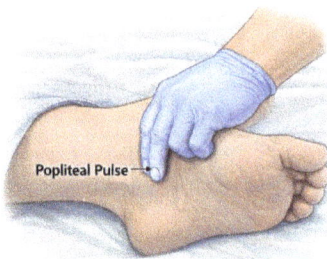

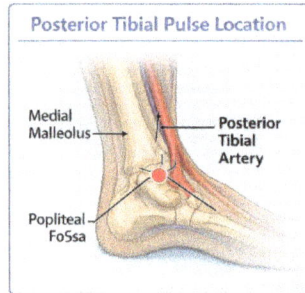

Posterior Tibial Pulse (Peripheral)

- Located behind and slightly below the medial malleolus (inner ankle bone)
- Useful for assessing peripheral circulation in the lower limb

Popliteal Pulse

Posterior Tibial Pulse Location

Medial Malleolus

Posterior Tibial Artery

Popliteal FoSsa

Dorsalis Pedis Pulse (Peripheral)

- Located on the dorsum (top) of the foot, lateral to the extensor hallucis longus tendon
- May be absent in some healthy individuals and should always be compared bilaterally[25]

Dorsalis Pedis Pulse (Peripheral)

- Located on the dorsum (top) of the foot, lateral to the extensor hallucis longus tendon
- May be absent in some healthy individuals and should be compared bilaterally[25]

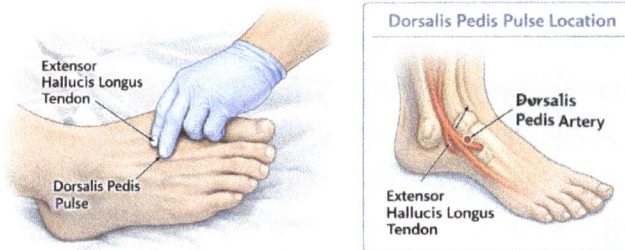

Dorsalis Pedis Pulse Location

Key Clinical Points

- In unresponsive adults, assess the carotid or femoral pulse
- In conscious patients, the radial pulse is usually sufficient
- Always assess the rate, rhythm, and strength of the pulse
- Absence of a peripheral pulse does not necessarily indicate cardiac arrest and should be interpreted alongside breathing and level of responsiveness

Pulse Oximeter

A pulse oximeter is a non-invasive fingertip device used to measure oxygen saturation (SpO_2) and pulse rate. Although it has no absolute contraindications, readings may be unreliable in cases of poor peripheral perfusion, movement, nail varnish or artificial nails, carbon monoxide exposure, severe anaemia, skin pigmentation, strong ambient light, or incorrect or faulty sensor placement. It should be used to support, not replace, clinical assessment.

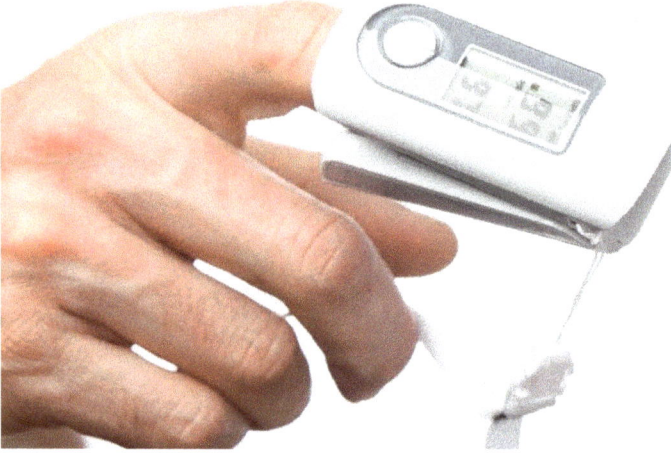

Blood Pressure Values (Adults)

Blood pressure (BP) is recorded as **systolic pressure over diastolic pressure** and is measured in millimetres of mercury (mmHg). Values should always be interpreted in the context of the patient's symptoms, clinical condition, and baseline readings.

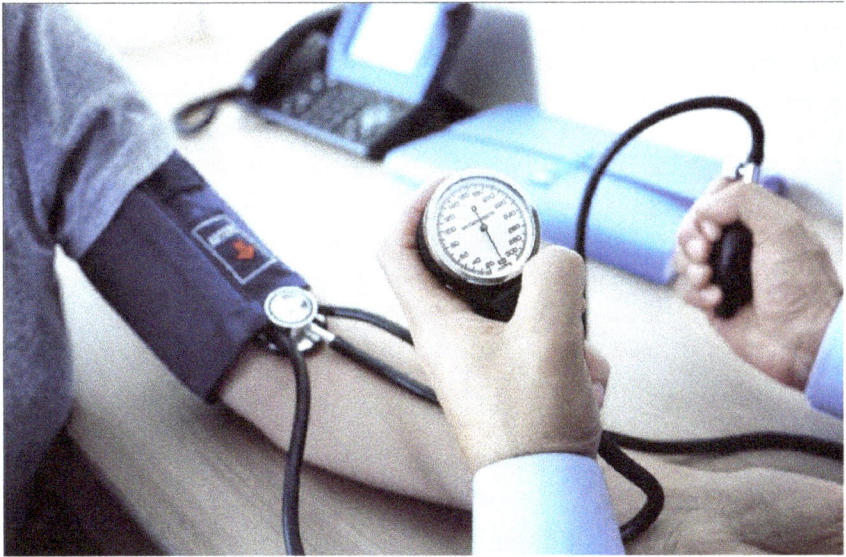

Normal Blood Pressure

- **Systolic: <120 mmHg**
- **Diastolic: <80 mmHg**

This range is associated with the lowest risk of cardiovascular disease in adults.[26]

Elevated Blood Pressure (High-Normal)

- **Systolic: 120–129 mmHg**
- **Diastolic: <80 mmHg**

Patients in this range are not classified as hypertensive but may require monitoring and lifestyle advice.[26]

Hypertension

Hypertension is diagnosed when blood pressure is **persistently elevated**:

- **Systolic: ≥140 mmHg**

- **Diastolic: ≥90 mmHg**

Diagnosis should be confirmed using repeated clinic readings, ambulatory blood pressure monitoring (ABPM), or home blood pressure monitoring (HBPM).[27]

Hypotension

- **Systolic: ≤90 mmHg**
- Often associated with symptoms such as dizziness, syncope, confusion, or signs of shock

Hypotension is clinically significant **when accompanied by symptoms or evidence of poor perfusion**, rather than by numerical value alone.[28]

Key Clinical Points for Practice

- Blood pressure should be interpreted alongside **pulse, respiratory rate, oxygen saturation, and level of consciousness**
- Sudden changes from a patient's normal baseline may indicate **acute illness or deterioration**
- In dental practice, **symptomatic hypotension or severe hypertension requires escalation and emergency referral**

Essential Cardiac Anatomy & Physiology

Structure of the heart

The heart is a **muscular, four-chambered organ** that pumps blood throughout the body. It is divided into **upper chambers (atria)** and **lower chambers (ventricles)**, with a central wall (septum) separating the right and left sides.

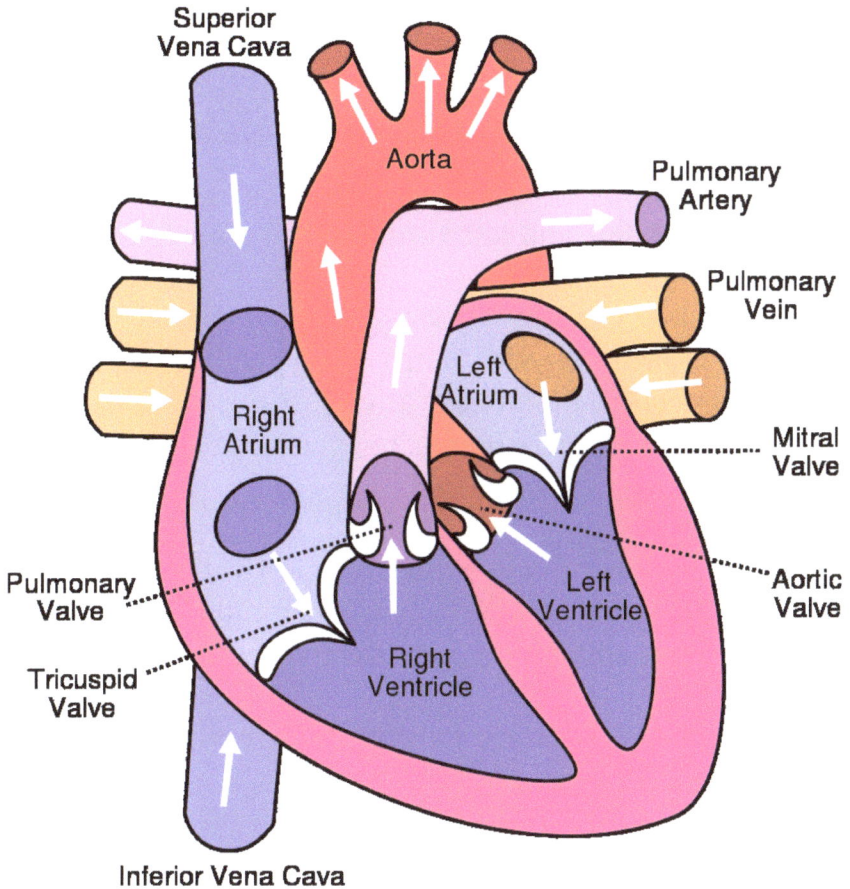

Upper Chambers – The Atria

The **right atrium** and **left atrium** are the two upper chambers of the heart.

- The **right atrium** receives **deoxygenated blood** returning from the body via the superior and inferior vena cava.
- The **left atrium** receives **oxygenated blood** from the lungs via the pulmonary veins.

The atria act as **receiving chambers**, collecting blood, and passing it into the ventricles below.

Lower Chambers – The Ventricles

The **right ventricle** and **left ventricle** are the two lower chambers of the heart.

- The **right ventricle** pumps deoxygenated blood to the lungs via the pulmonary artery for oxygenation.
- The **left ventricle** pumps oxygenated blood to the rest of the body via the aorta.

The ventricles have **thicker muscular walls** than the atria, especially the left ventricle, because they must generate enough force to circulate blood effectively.

The Septum

The **septum** is a strong muscular wall that separates the **right side** of the heart from the **left side**.

- It prevents the mixing of **oxygenated and deoxygenated blood**

- It ensures efficient circulation and oxygen delivery to the body

Clinical relevance (BLS context):

Understanding heart structure helps explain how cardiac arrest disrupts circulation and why **effective chest compressions** are vital to manually pump blood from the ventricles to the brain and vital organs.

4.2 Blood vessels

- **Arteries** carry blood away from the heart (usually oxygenated, except pulmonary artery).
- **Veins** return blood to the heart (usually deoxygenated, except pulmonary veins).
- **Capillaries** enable gas/nutrient exchange.

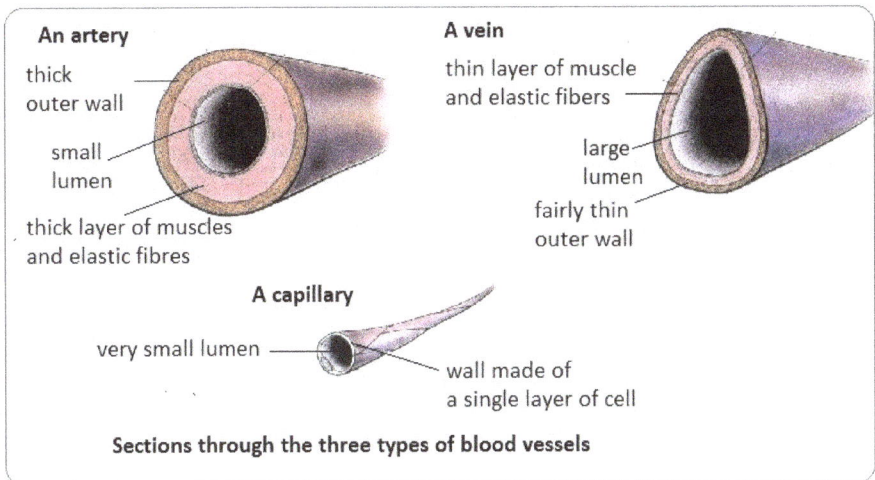

An artery
thick outer wall
small lumen
thick layer of muscles and elastic fibres

A vein
thin layer of muscle and elastic fibers
large lumen
fairly thin outer wall

A capillary
very small lumen
wall made of a single layer of cell

Sections through the three types of blood vessels

4.3 Valves

Right side:

- **Tricuspid valve** (RA → RV)
- **Pulmonary valve** (RV → pulmonary artery)

Left side:

- **Mitral valve** (LA → LV)
- **Aortic valve** (LV → aorta)

Heart Valves

Heart valves ensure **one-way blood flow** through the heart by opening and closing with pressure changes during each heartbeat.

Right side (deoxygenated blood):

- **Tricuspid valve** – allows blood flow from the **right atrium (RA) to right ventricle (RV)**
- **Pulmonary valve** – allows blood flow from the **right ventricle to the pulmonary artery**

Left side (oxygenated blood):

- **Mitral valve** – allows blood flow from the **left atrium (LA) to left ventricle (LV)**
- **Aortic valve** – allows blood flow from the **left ventricle to the aorta**

Key point: Valves prevent backflow and ensure efficient circulation, which is essential for effective blood flow during normal heart function and CPR.

4.4 Electrical conduction

Components of the Heart's Electrical Conduction System

The heart's electrical conduction system controls the **rate and rhythm of the heartbeat**, ensuring coordinated contraction of the atria and ventricles.

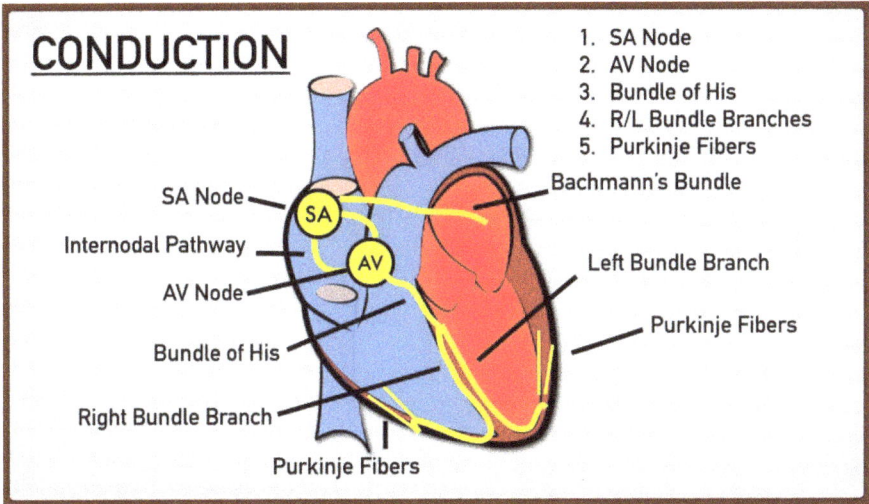

CONDUCTION

1. SA Node
2. AV Node
3. Bundle of His
4. R/L Bundle Branches
5. Purkinje Fibers

SA Node
Internodal Pathway
AV Node
Bundle of His
Right Bundle Branch
Purkinje Fibers

Bachmann's Bundle
Left Bundle Branch
Purkinje Fibers

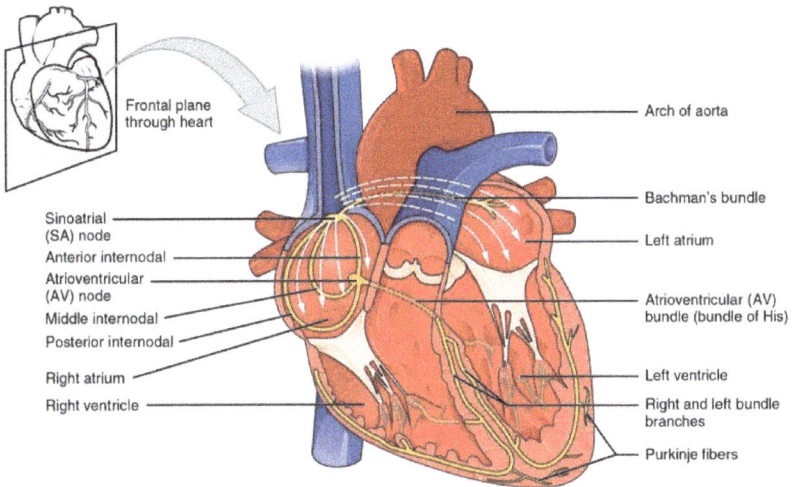

Frontal plane through heart

Arch of aorta

Bachman's bundle

Sinoatrial (SA) node
Anterior internodal
Atrioventricular (AV) node
Middle internodal
Posterior internodal
Right atrium
Right ventricle

Left atrium
Atrioventricular (AV) bundle (bundle of His)
Left ventricle
Right and left bundle branches
Purkinje fibers

Anterior view of frontal section

Sinoatrial (SA) Node – Natural Pacemaker

- Located in the **right atrium**
- Initiates each heartbeat by generating electrical impulses
- Sets the normal heart rate (usually **60–100 beats per minute** in adults)

Atrioventricular (AV) Node

- Located between the atria and ventricles
- Delays the electrical impulse briefly, allowing the ventricles time to fill with blood
- Acts as a protective gatekeeper, controlling impulse transmission

Bundle of His (Atrioventricular Bundle)

- Conducts electrical impulses from the AV node into the ventricles
- Splits into right and left bundle branches along the interventricular septum

Purkinje Fibres

- Fine network of fibres spreading throughout the ventricular muscle
- Rapidly distributes electrical impulses
- Causes the ventricles to contract together, producing an effective heartbeat

Clinical relevance (BLS context):
Disruption of this conduction system can lead to **life-threatening arrhythmias**. During cardiac arrest, CPR and

defibrillation aim to restore organised electrical activity and effective circulation.

Acute Coronary Syndrome

Suspected heart attack / cardiac-sounding chest pain:

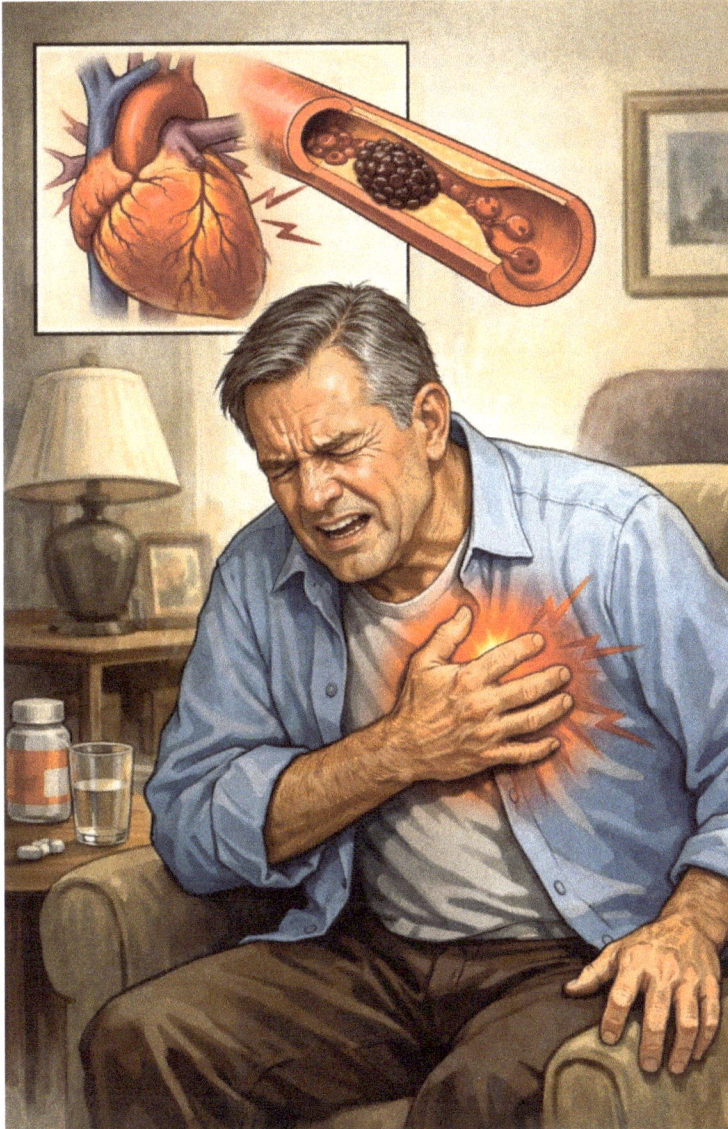

A heart attack (myocardial infarction) is usually caused by reduced or blocked blood flow in a coronary artery, leading to heart muscle damage. Rapid action reduces death and complications.

Recognise a heart attack

Common features include:

- Central **chest pain/pressure/tightness** (may radiate to arm, jaw, neck, back)
- **Breathlessness**
- **Sweating**, pale/clammy skin
- **Nausea/vomiting**, dizziness, collapse
- Anxiety or a "sense of impending doom"

What to do (step-by-step)

1. **Call 999/112 immediately** (do not delay). (Resuscitation Council UK)
2. **Position for comfort**: sit or lie them in a comfortable position (many prefer semi-sitting). Reassure and keep them still. (Resuscitation Council UK)
3. **Aspirin 300 mg (adults)**: encourage and assist the person to **self-administer 300 mg aspirin** as soon as possible **unless contraindicated** (at minimum: **do not give if known aspirin allergy**; follow local policy/PGD for other contraindications). Chewable or dissolvable is preferred. (Resuscitation Council UK)

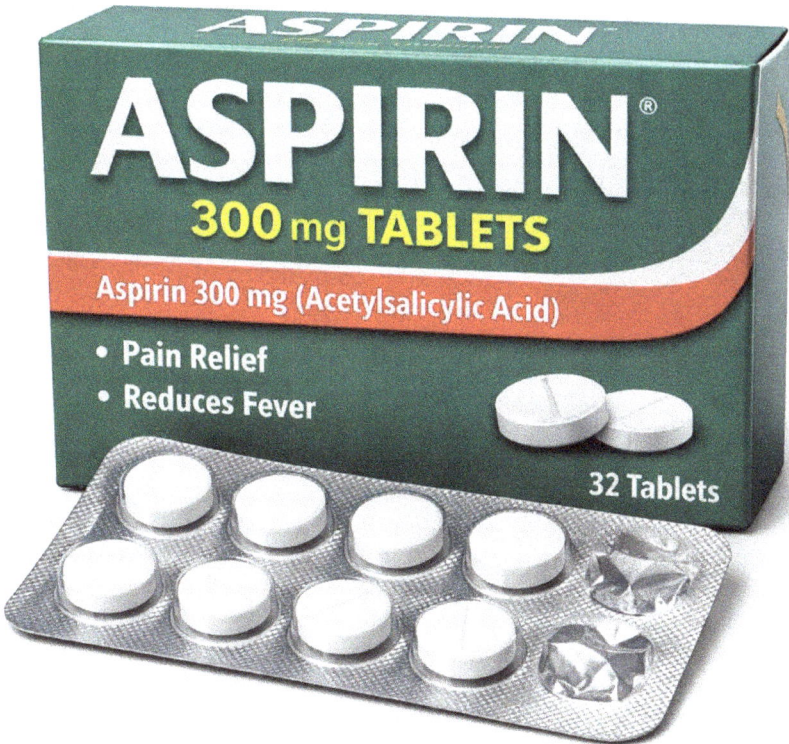

4. **If they have known angina**: assist them to **self-administer their GTN (nitroglycerine) spray/tablets**. ([Resuscitation Council UK](#))
5. **Stay with them and monitor** continuously:
   - ○ If they become **unresponsive** and are **not breathing normally**, start **CPR** and use an **AED** as soon as available. ([Resuscitation Council UK](#))

Key safety notes (good practice)

- Do **not** let them drive themselves to hospital.
- If symptoms worsen, or they develop reduced consciousness, treat as time-critical and escalate urgently (999/112 or local emergency response).
- In healthcare settings, follow local pathways for ECG, oxygen titration if hypoxic, and rapid transfer for reperfusion where indicated (per NICE ACS guidance). (NICE)

5.4 Angina

Angina is chest discomfort resulting from transient myocardial ischaemia caused by an imbalance between myocardial oxygen supply and demand.

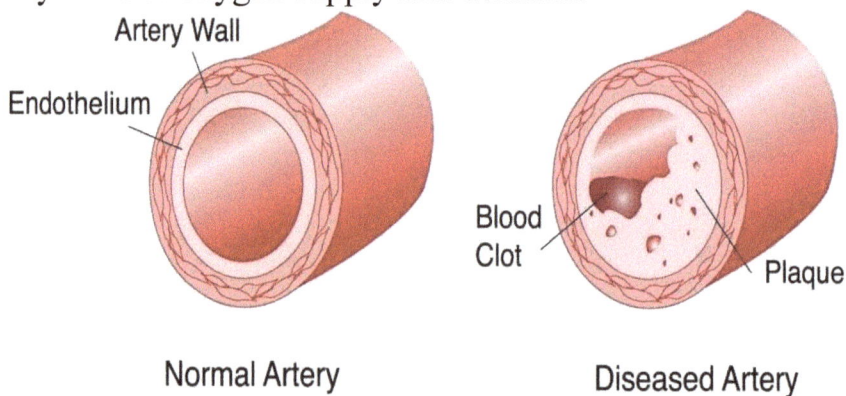

Normal Artery   Diseased Artery

- **Stable angina:** Predictable chest discomfort precipitated by physical exertion or emotional stress, relieved by rest and/or glyceryl trinitrate (GTN).
- **Unstable angina:** New-onset angina, crescendo (worsening) angina, or angina occurring at rest. This is classified as an acute coronary syndrome and requires urgent assessment and management.

GTN safety note: GTN should not be administered in patients with hypotension. In UK practice, GTN is contraindicated if systolic blood pressure is ≤90 mmHg; always follow local trust or ambulance service protocols.

How to use GTN (glyceryl trinitrate) **for angina**

How to use GTN (glyceryl trinitrate) for angina

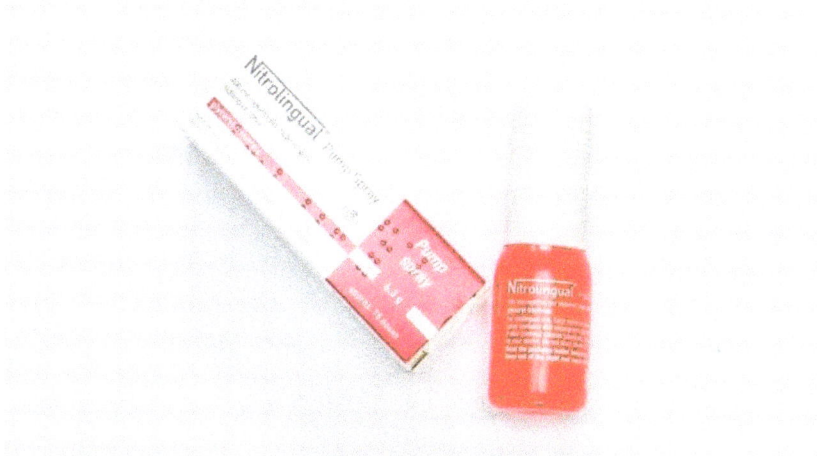

1) When to use

- At the **onset of chest pain** suggestive of angina
- **Prophylactically** 5–10 minutes before predictable exertion (e.g. climbing stairs), if advised

2) Position & preparation

- **Sit or lie down** (GTN can cause dizziness or a sudden drop in blood pressure)
- If using a **spray**, remove the cap and hold the bottle upright
- If using **tablets**, ensure they are fresh and not expired

3) Administration

Sublingual spray

- Spray **1 dose under the tongue**
- Do **not inhale**
- Close mouth; do not swallow immediately

Sublingual tablet

- Place **1 tablet under the tongue**
- Allow it to dissolve completely
- Do **not** chew or swallow

4) Reassessment

- Relief should occur within **1–5 minutes**
- If pain persists, you may **repeat every 5 minutes**, up to **3 doses total** (unless told otherwise)

5) When to seek urgent help

- **No relief after 5 minutes** of the first dose → **call emergency services**
- Chest pain lasting **>15 minutes**, worsening pain, or pain at rest

6) Common effects (expected)

- Headache, flushing
- Light-headedness or dizziness
  (These indicate the drug is working but still requires caution.)

7) Safety points (important)

- **Do not use if hypotensive** — follow local protocol (in the UK, avoid if **SBP ≤90 mmHg**)
- **Do not combine with PDE-5 inhibitors** (e.g. sildenafil/Viagra) within the last **24–48 hours**
- Store tablets in the **original glass container**; once opened, they lose potency over time

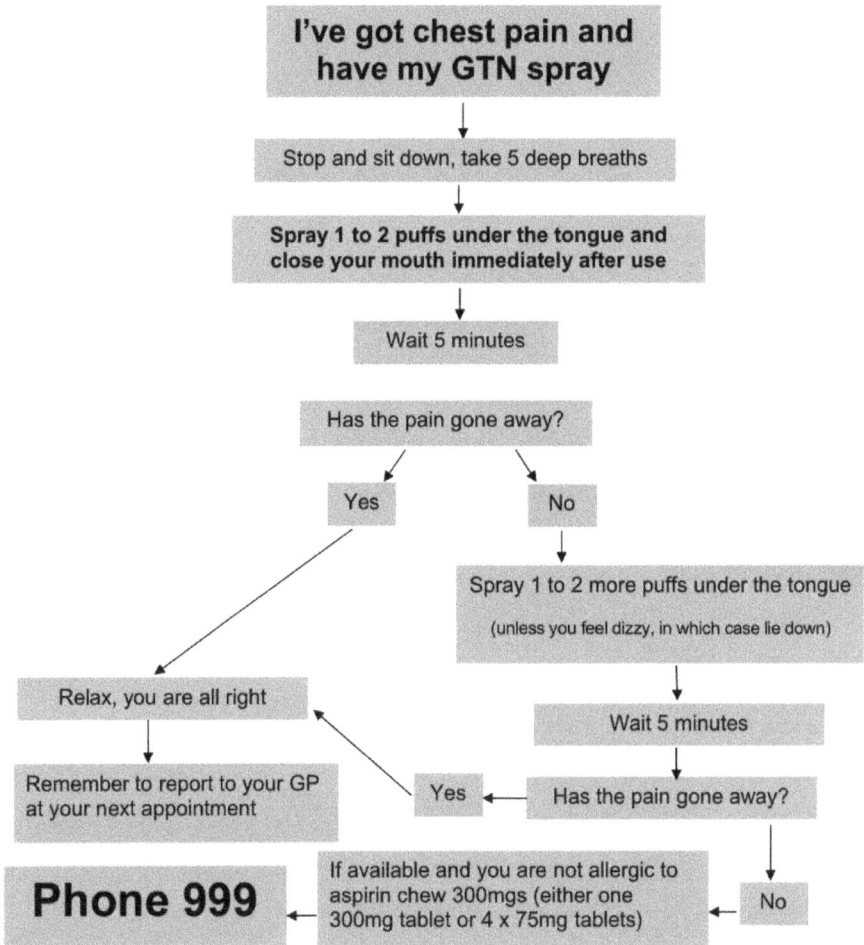

I've got chest pain and have my GTN spray

Stop and sit down, take 5 deep breaths

Spray 1 to 2 puffs under the tongue and close your mouth immediately after use

Wait 5 minutes

Has the pain gone away?

Yes

No

Spray 1 to 2 more puffs under the tongue

(unless you feel dizzy, in which case lie down)

Relax, you are all right

Remember to report to your GP at your next appointment

Wait 5 minutes

Yes

Has the pain gone away?

Phone 999

If available and you are not allergic to aspirin chew 300mgs (either one 300mg tablet or 4 x 75mg tablets)

No

Chapter 6 — Cardiac arrest rhythms

What is a cardiac arrest?

Key definition

Cardiac arrest is the sudden loss of effective cardiac output, resulting in loss of consciousness and absence of normal breathing, requiring immediate cardiopulmonary resuscitation and defibrillation where indicated.

What happens in cardiac arrest?

- The heart **stops pumping blood effectively**
- The person becomes:
  - **Unresponsive**
  - **Not breathing normally** (or only gasping)
  - **Pulseless**
- **Loss of consciousness** occurs within seconds
- **Irreversible brain injury** can begin within 3–5 minutes without intervention

Cardiac arrest vs heart attack (important distinction)

Cardiac arrest	Heart attack (myocardial infarction)
Electrical/mechanical failure	Circulatory problem (blocked coronary artery)
Collapse	Chest pain common
No pulse	Pulse usually present
Immediate CPR/defib required	Urgent medical treatment

A **heart attack can cause a cardiac arrest**, but they are not the same.

Cardiac arrest rhythms

Shockable vs Non-shockable rhythms

In cardiac arrest, rhythms are divided based on **whether defibrillation can correct the underlying electrical problem**.

Shockable rhythms

Rhythms:

- **Ventricular fibrillation (VF)**
- **Pulseless ventricular tachycardia (VT)**

What is happening physiologically:

- The heart has **chaotic or excessively fast electrical activity**
- There is **no effective cardiac output**, despite electrical activity
- The myocardium is electrically active but **disorganised**

AED / defibrillation principle:

- An **AED may advise a shock**
- Defibrillation delivers a high-energy shock to:
  - Stop all electrical activity momentarily
  - Allow the sinoatrial (SA) node to restart a **perfusing rhythm**
- **Early defibrillation is critical** — survival decreases by ~7–10% per minute without it

Key BLS message:

Shockable rhythms = electricity problem → **defibrillation + CPR**

Non-shockable rhythms

Rhythms:

- **Asystole** (flatline)
- **Pulseless electrical activity (PEA)**

What is happening physiologically:

- **Asystole:** No electrical activity → no contraction
- **PEA:** Organised electrical activity but **no mechanical output**
- The problem is usually **metabolic, hypoxic, or obstructive**, not electrical

AED / defibrillation principle:

- **AED will NOT advise a shock**
- Defibrillation is ineffective because there is:
- No chaotic electrical activity to reset

Management focus:

- **High-quality CPR**
- **Early adrenaline (ALS)**
- **Identify and treat reversible causes**

Non-shockable rhythms = circulation/physiology problem. Treatment-**CPR + cause correction**

Cardiac arrest is diagnosed clinically and then classified by rhythm:

Ventricular fibrillation (VF) —

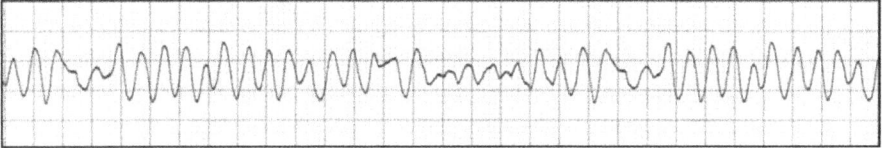

Ventricular Fibrillation (V-fib)

Rhythm: Chaotic
Rate: Chaotic
P Waves: Absent
P-R Interval: Absent
QRS: Absent

Clinical Significance: Ventricular fibrillation is lethal with no cardiac output. Defibrillate with an initial unsynchronized dose of 360 joules monophasic or 120-200 joules biphasic. 1mg Ephinephrine 1:10,000 is the drug of choice given every 3-5 minutes.

Definition:
Ventricular fibrillation is a **cardiac arrest rhythm** caused by **chaotic, disorganised ventricular electrical activity**, resulting in **no effective cardiac output**.

ECG features:

- No identifiable P waves, QRS complexes, or T waves
- Irregular, chaotic waveform
- Variable amplitude (coarse or fine VF)

Clinical features:

- Unconscious
- Not breathing normally
- Pulseless

Management:

- Immediate **CPR**
- **Early defibrillation** (shockable rhythm)

49

Key point:

VF = electrical chaos → **defibrillate immediately**.

Pulseless Ventricular Tachycardia (pVT)

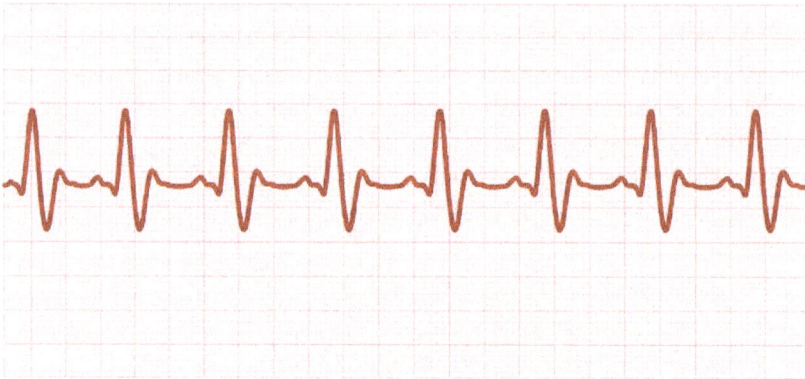

Pulseless Ventricular Tachycardia (pVT)

Pulseless ventricular tachycardia is a **life-threatening cardiac arrest rhythm**. It occurs when the ventricles beat amazingly fast due to abnormal electrical activity, but **the heart does not pump blood effectively**, so **no pulse is present**.

Key features

- **Origin:** Ventricles
- **Heart rate:** Usually >150–250 beats/min
- **Pulse:** Absent

- **Patient state:** Unconscious, not breathing normally
- **ECG appearance:**
  - Wide QRS complexes (>120 ms)
  - Regular, rapid rhythm
  - No visible P waves
  - Can be **monomorphic** (uniform shape) or **polymorphic**

Why there is no pulse

Although the heart is electrically active, the ventricles contract so rapidly and inefficiently that **cardiac output is zero**, resulting in circulatory collapse.

Common causes

- Acute myocardial infarction (ischemia)
- Hypoxia
- Electrolyte abnormalities ($\downarrow K^+$, $\downarrow Mg^{2+}$)
- Drug toxicity (e.g., antiarrhythmics)
- Structural heart disease

Management (ACLS)

Pulseless VT is treated **the same as ventricular fibrillation**:

1. **Immediate CPR**
2. **Early defibrillation (unsynchronised shock)**
3. **Adrenaline**
4. **Amiodarone**
5. Identify and treat **reversible causes (Hs & Ts)**

Important: pVT is a **shockable rhythm**. Delay in defibrillation significantly reduces survival.

Non-shockable:

Asystole

Asystole is a **cardiac arrest rhythm** characterized by a **complete absence of electrical activity in the heart**. It is commonly referred to as a **"flatline."**

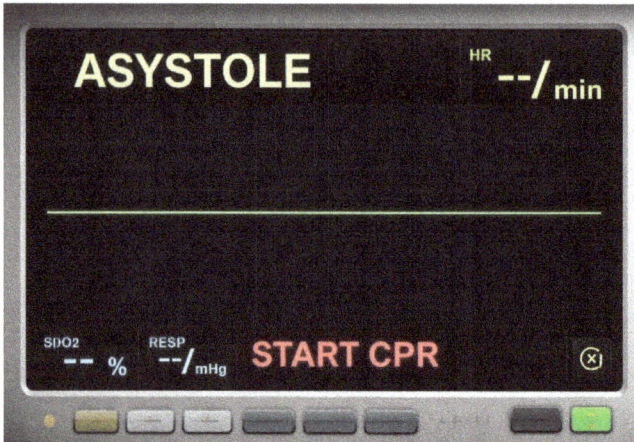

Key features

- **Electrical activity:** None
- **Pulse:** Absent
- **Heart rate:** 0
- **Patient state:** Unconscious, apnoeic, or agonal breathing
- **ECG appearance:**
  - Flat or flat line
  - No P waves
  - No QRS complexes
  - No T waves

Pathophysiology

Asystole occurs when the heart's electrical system completely fails. Without electrical impulses, the myocardium does not contract, resulting in **no cardiac output and no circulation**.

Common causes

Often associated with prolonged hypoxia or severe systemic illness:

- Hypoxia
- Severe acidosis
- Hypothermia
- Hyperkalemia
- Massive myocardial infarction
- Drug overdose or poisoning
- Prolonged untreated cardiac arrest

(These are part of the **Hs and Ts** in ACLS.)

Management

Asystole is a **non-shockable rhythm**.

1. **Immediate high-quality CPR**
2. **Adrenaline** every 3–5 minutes
3. **Airway management and oxygen**
4. Identify and treat **reversible causes (Hs & Ts)**

Defibrillation is NOT indicated in asystole because there is no electrical activity to reset.

Pulseless electrical activity (PEA)

Pulseless electrical activity (PEA) is a **cardiac arrest rhythm** in which **organised electrical activity is seen on the ECG, but there is no palpable pulse**.

Pulseless Electrical
Activity (PEA)

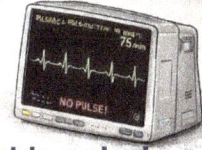

Organised electrical rhythm but <u>NO</u> palpable pulse!

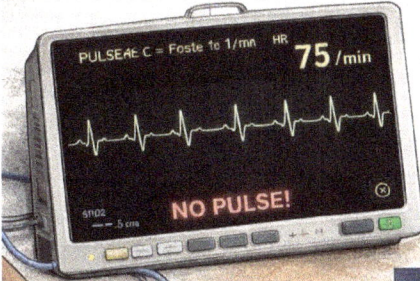

✅ **Organised ECG rhythm**

❌ **No pulse**

⚠️ **Not a shockable rhythm**

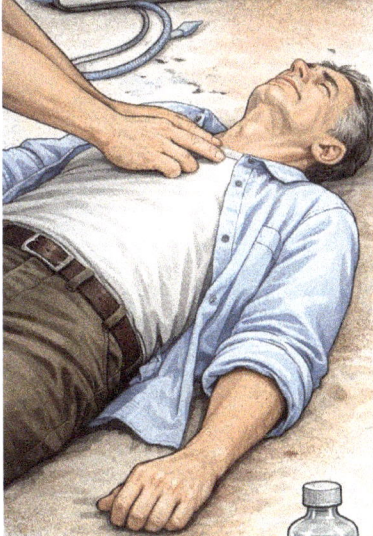

Common Causes (Hs & Ts):

- **Hypovolaemia**
- **Hypoxia**
- **Acidosis**
- **Electrolytes**
- **Hypothermia**
- **Tension pneumothorax**
- **Tamponade**
- **Toxins**
- **Thrombosis**

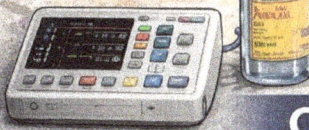

CPR + Treat the cause!

- **ECG:** Organised rhythm (may look normal)
- **Pulse:** Absent
- **Shockable:** No
- **Cause:** Usually due to **reversible conditions**, not an electrical problem

Common causes (Hs & Ts):
Hypovolemia, Hypoxia, Acidosis, Electrolyte imbalance, Hypothermia, Tension pneumothorax, Tamponade, Toxins, Thrombosis, Trauma

Management:
Immediate **CPR**, **adrenaline**, airway/oxygen, and **treat the underlying cause**.

Always assess the **patient, not just the monitor**.

Causes of cardiac arrest

Common causes include:

- Acute coronary syndrome
- Severe hypoxia
- Electrolyte disturbances
- Massive haemorrhage
- Tension pneumothorax
- Drug toxicity
  *(summarised as the **4 Hs & 4 Ts**)*

Causes of cardiac arrest: the "4 Hs & 4 Ts"

The 4 Hs

1. Hypoxia

Meaning: Inadequate oxygen delivery to tissues

Examples:

- Airway obstruction
- Respiratory failure
- Severe asthma or pneumonia

Why it causes arrest:

- Myocardium becomes ischaemic → electrical failure

Treatment focus:

- Airway management
- High-flow oxygen
- Ventilation

2. Hypovolaemia

Meaning: Critically reduced circulating blood volume

Examples:

- Massive haemorrhage (trauma, GI bleed)
- Severe dehydration

Why it causes arrest:

- Insufficient preload → no cardiac output

Treatment focus:

- Control bleeding
- Rapid IV fluids / blood products

3. Hypo- or hyperkalaemia (and metabolic causes)

Meaning: Dangerous electrolyte or metabolic disturbances

Examples:

- Renal failure
- DKA
- Severe acidosis

Why it causes arrest:

- Disrupts myocardial electrical conduction

Treatment focus:

- Calcium, insulin/glucose, bicarbonate (ALS)
- Correct underlying cause

4. Hypothermia

Meaning: Core temperature <35°C

Why it causes arrest:

- Depresses myocardial function
- Increases arrhythmia risk

Treatment focus:

- Gentle handling
- Active rewarming
- Prolonged resuscitation if indicated
  (*"Not dead until warm and dead"*)

The 4 Ts

1. Tension pneumothorax

Meaning: Air trapped under pressure in the pleural space

Why it causes arrest:

- Compresses lungs and great vessels
- Reduces venous return and cardiac output

Treatment focus:

- Immediate needle decompression
- Chest drain

2. Cardiac tamponade

Meaning: Fluid accumulation in the pericardial sac

Why it causes arrest:

- Prevents ventricular filling

Treatment focus:

- Pericardiocentesis
- Treat underlying cause (e.g. trauma)

3. Toxins

Meaning: Drug or chemical poisoning

Examples:

- Opioids

- Beta-blockers
- Tricyclic antidepressants

Why it causes arrest:

- Direct myocardial depression or arrhythmias

Treatment focus:

- Antidotes (e.g. naloxone)
- Supportive care

4. Thrombosis (coronary or pulmonary)

Meaning:

- **Coronary thrombosis:** Acute myocardial infarction
- **Pulmonary thrombosis:** Massive pulmonary embolism

Why it causes arrest:

- Sudden loss of effective circulation

Treatment focus:

- PCI / thrombolysis
- Advanced life support

AIRWAY MANAGEMENT

OROPHARYNGEAL AIRWAY

Why OPA sizing matters

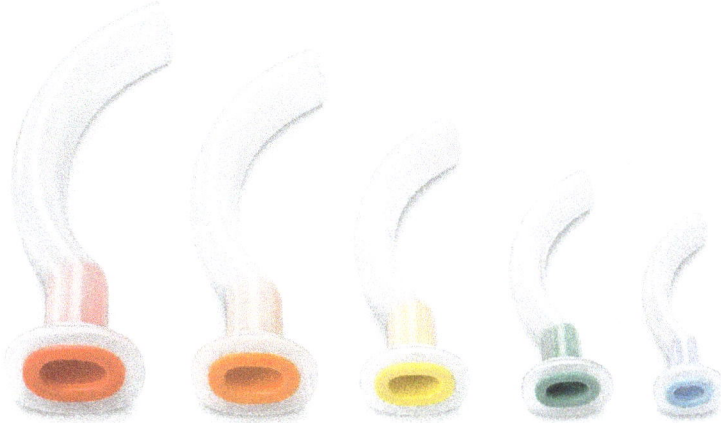

Choosing the right size of the OPA matters because the wrong size can obstruct the airway or cause injury:

Too small: Pushes the tongue backwards, worsening obstruction

Too large: presses on the epiglottis, gagging, trauma, vomiting

Correct size: keeps the airway open, allows ventilation, and allows effective airway management

THE SIZING METHODS

Corner of the mouth to the angle of the Jaw

Or from incisors to the earlobe

INSERTING THE OPA

OPA insertion: step-by-step

1) Confirm it is appropriate

- Use an OPA **only in an unconscious patient** with **no gag reflex** (or deeply reduced reflexes).
- If the patient is conscious/has a gag reflex → consider an **NPA** instead (if not contraindicated).

2) Prepare and position

- Call for help if needed; apply standard precautions.
- Position the patient:
  - **Head-tilt chin-lift** (if no trauma suspected), or
  - **Jaw thrust** (if trauma suspected).
- Suction the mouth if there are secretions/vomit.

3) Choose the correct size

- Measure from the **corner of the mouth to the angle of the jaw** (or earlobe/tragus, depending on local teaching).
- Correct size helps avoid pushing the tongue back or causing obstruction.

4) Open the mouth and insert

Adults (common method):

1. Open the mouth using a scissor technique (thumb on lower teeth/gum, index on upper).
2. Insert the OPA **upside down** (curve facing upward) along the hard palate.
3. Advance until the tip reaches the soft palate.
4. **Rotate 180°** so the curve follows the tongue.
5. Advance gently until the **flange rests on the lips/teeth**.

Alternative method (often used in children / to reduce trauma):

- Insert the OPA **the right way up** using a **tongue depressor** to hold the tongue forward, then advance gently until seated.

5) Confirm it is working

- Look/listen/feel for improved airflow.
- Check for effective chest rise with ventilation if you are bagging.
- Monitor oxygen saturation, breathing pattern, and airway sounds.

6) Secure and reassess continuously

- Keep the airway in place only while it is tolerated and effective.
- Reassess frequently: airway patency, oxygenation, and need for suction.

- If gagging/vomiting occurs, **remove the OPA** and manage the airway (reposition/suction; consider alternative adjunct).

Key safety points

- Never force it—use gentle technique.
- Wrong size can worsen obstruction.
- OPAs do **not** protect against aspiration—use suction and appropriate positioning.

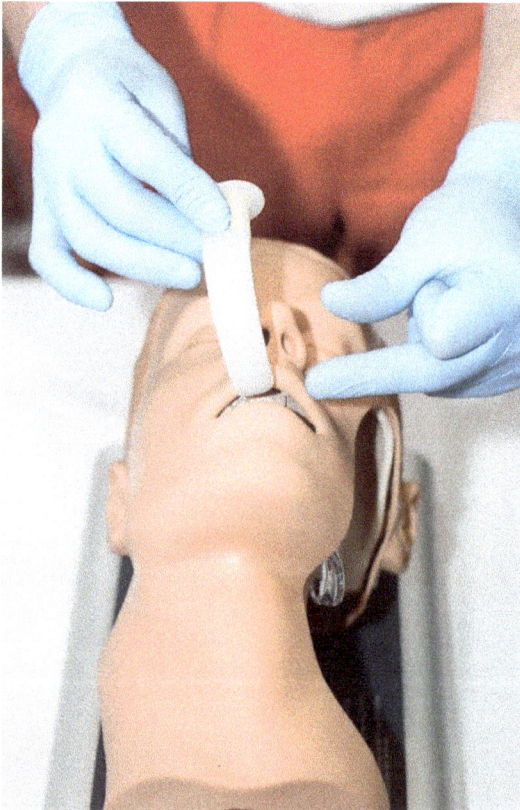

CARDIOPULMONARY RESUSCITATION (CPR)

Core Principles of CPR (All Ages)

- Ensure the **safety** of the rescuer and the casualty
- **Early recognition** of cardiac arrest
- **Early CPR**
- **Early defibrillation**
- **Early advanced care**

If unresponsive and not breathing normally → start CPR immediately and send for a defibrillator.

ADULT CPR

Ensure the scene is safe for you and the casualty.

CHECK IF THE PATIENT IS RESPONSIVE

Kneel beside him.

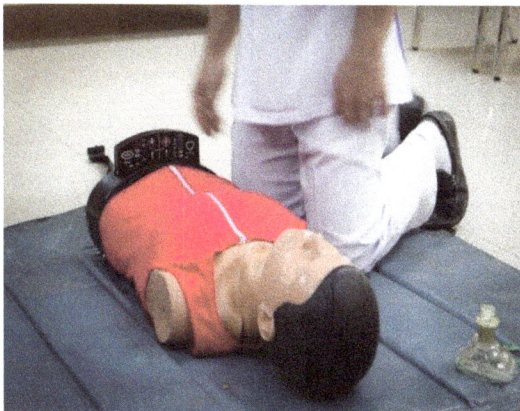

SHAKE THE PATIENT'S SHOULDER OR SQUEEZE THE EARLOBES OR THE TRAPEZIUS MUSCLES

Check whether the casualty is responsive by shaking the casualty's shoulder, speaking to the casualty, and saying, "Wake up!" "Squeeze my hand, squeeze the ear lobes, or press the supraorbital notch or the trapezius

muscle.

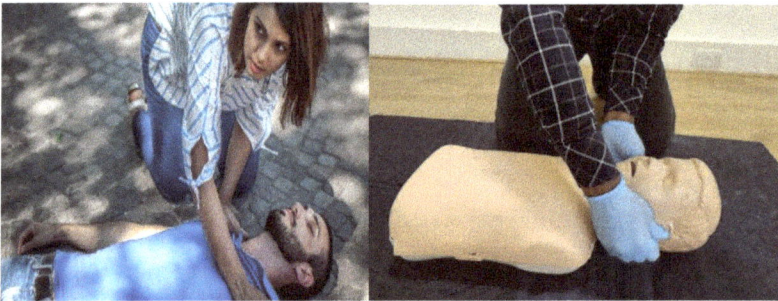

CALL 999/112 OR ASK A BYSTANDER TO CALL IF THE PATIENT IS UNRESPONSIVE. CALL 2222 IF IN THE HOSPITAL.

If unresponsive, proceed immediately to emergency call. Call first before checking breathing; call handlers will assist with breathing assessment.

☐ Ask for an **ambulance and AED**.

☐ If alone, use hands-free speaker or phone headset.

☐ Dispatchers will help assess and guide CPR.

Give your location, your name, the names of the casualty, and the patient's condition. Ask for oxygen, a defibrillator, and any other resources you require to assist you in conducting adequate resuscitation.

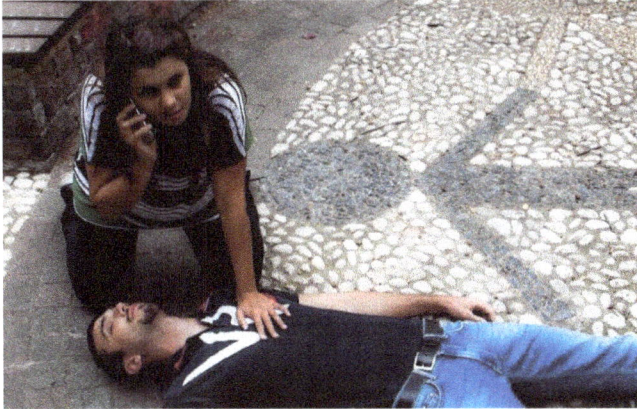

Place one hand on the forehead.

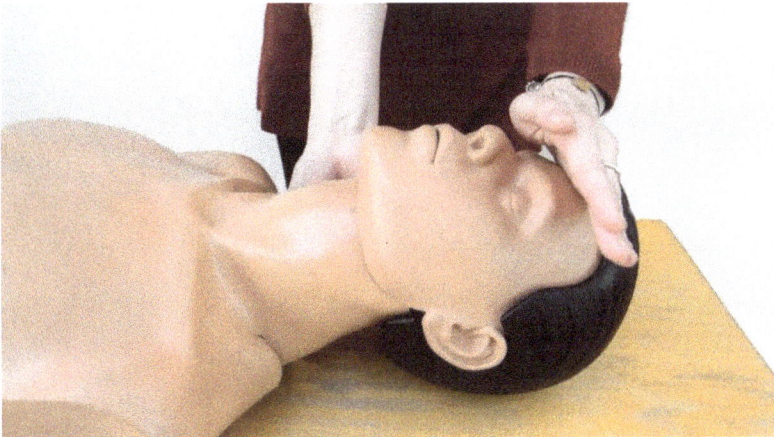

DO A HEAD TILT, CHIN LIFT

To maintain a clear airway, do a head tilt and chin lift. This will elevate the patient's relaxed tongue from the back of the airway to the front of the mouth. To achieve this, place your hand on your forehead, then lift your chin with the other hand.

ASSESS BREATHING

- Lower your head close to the casualty's face with your cheek close to the nose so that you can listen for any breath from the casualty's nose, feel the air from the casualty's nose on your cheek, and see the casualty's chest rise and fall. Do this for no more than 10 seconds. If the Casualty is **not breathing normally**, or breathing is **abnormal (agonal gasps)** assume cardiac arrest.
- **Do NOT delay CPR by over-analysing breathing patterns**.

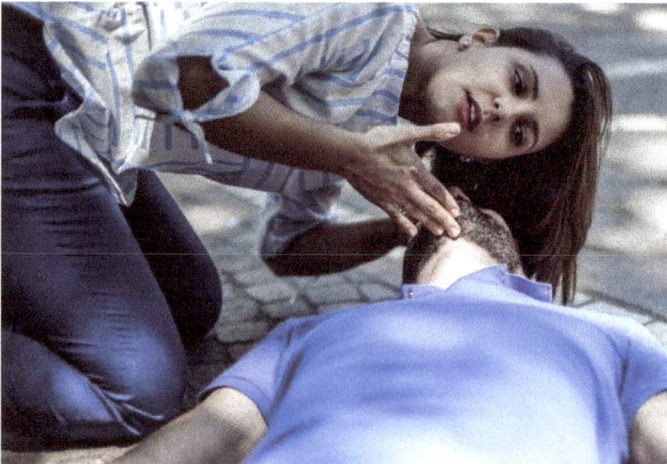

Start CPR Immediately

Chest Compressions

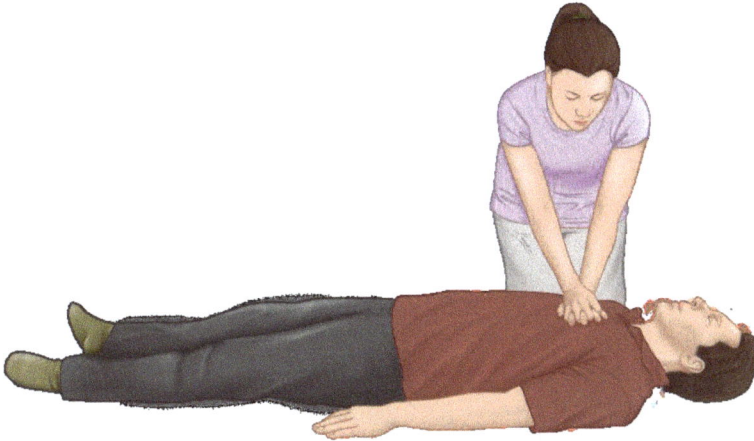

- Hand position: **centre of chest**
- Interlock fingers
- Arms straight, shoulders over hands
- Depth: **5–6 cm**
- Rate: **100–120 per minute**
- Allow **full chest recoil**

Compression–Ventilation Ratio

Conduct chest compressions immediately. For an adult, the ratio of compressions to breath should be thirty to two rescue breaths at 100-120 compressions per minute. On average, you are giving two compressions per second.

- **30 compressions: 2 breaths**

.

Minimise interruptions

Continue until professional help arrives or AED prompts otherwise.

- Place the heel of your hand in the centre of the patient's Chest slightly above the tip of the breastbone. The position of your hand on the chest is vital to effective CPR.
- Place the second hand on top of the first hand, which is already positioned on the chest. Interlock your fingers and give thirty compressions at a rate of two compressions per second.
- 100-120 compressions per minute. Make sure your arms are straight and leaning slightly over the patient.
- Press down on the casualty's chest to a depth of 5-6cm.
- Release your pressure on the chest and watch it recoil before pressing down on the chest again.

Rescue breaths

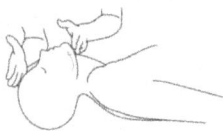

Open airways by lifting the chin slightly

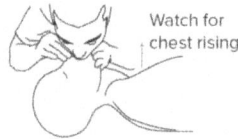

Watch for chest rising

Pinch nose and give two rescue breaths

Rescue Breaths

- **If trained and willing**:
  30 compressions : 2 breaths.
- **If untrained or unwilling to give breaths**:
  Continue **chest-compression-only CPR** guided by dispatcher.

Rescue Breath-Mouth-to-Mouth.

Rescue breaths may be delivered using mouth-to-mouth-and-nose or via a bag-valve-mask, ensuring an effective seal.

Seal your mouth over the patient's mouth while pinching their nose with your fingers. Keep the head tilted back to maintain an open airway. Only give mouth-to-mouth if you are confident there is no infection risk to you or the patient; if unsure, perform compression-only **CPR**. Give **two rescue breaths**, each lasting about **one second**. If you are unwilling or unable to give breaths, continue with **compression-only CPR**.

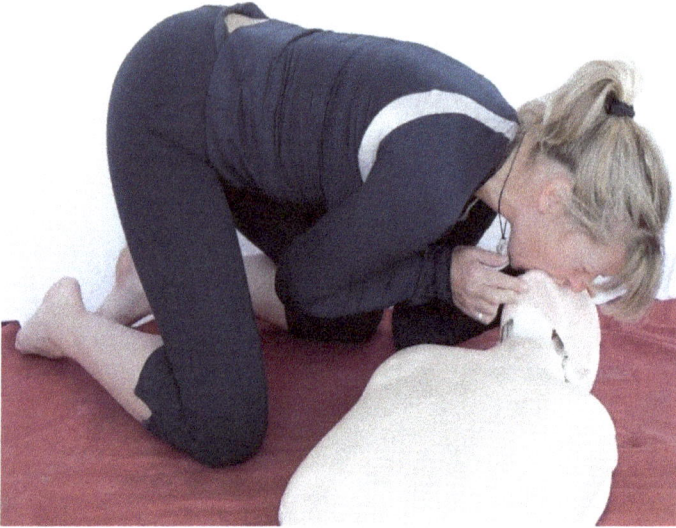

Rescue Breath-Mouth to face shield.

If you have a face shield, use it to minimise the risk of infection for you or the patient.

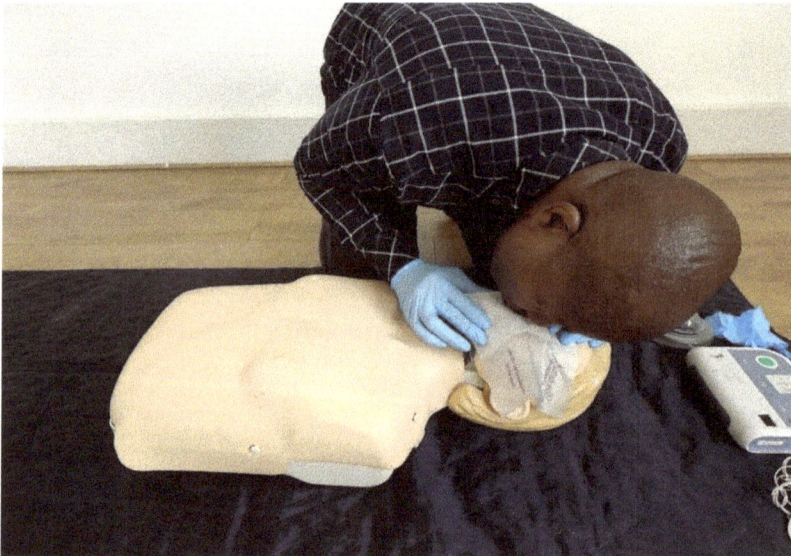

Rescue Breath- Mouth-to-Pocket Mask

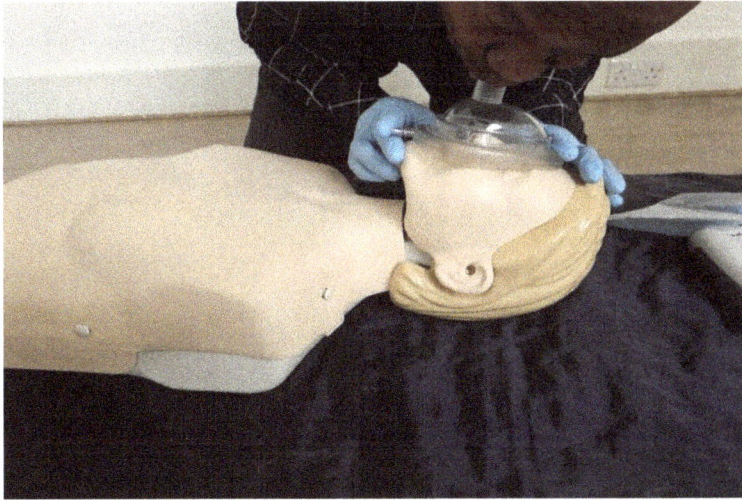

Rescue breathing can also be administered through a pocket Mask. This is another way of minimising the risk of infection.

Rescue Breath

Mouth-to-Bag Valve Mask (One-Person Technique)

One or two helpers can use a bag-valve mask (BVM). For a single-helpers technique, place one hand in a C-shape to seal the mask and use the other hand in an E-shape to maintain head tilt. Squeeze the bag to deliver breaths.

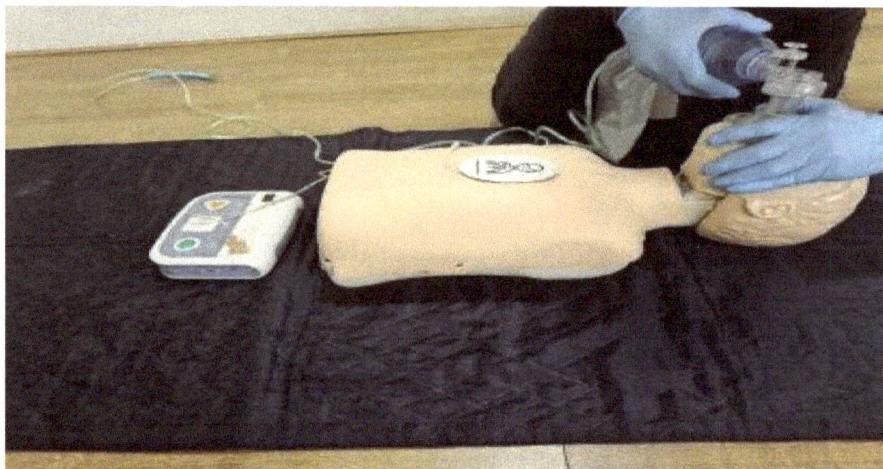

Mouth-to-Bag Valve Mask—Two Persons Technique.

With both hands, one helper seals the BVM mask over the patient's nose and mouth while the other helper presses the oxygen bag to release the oxygen.

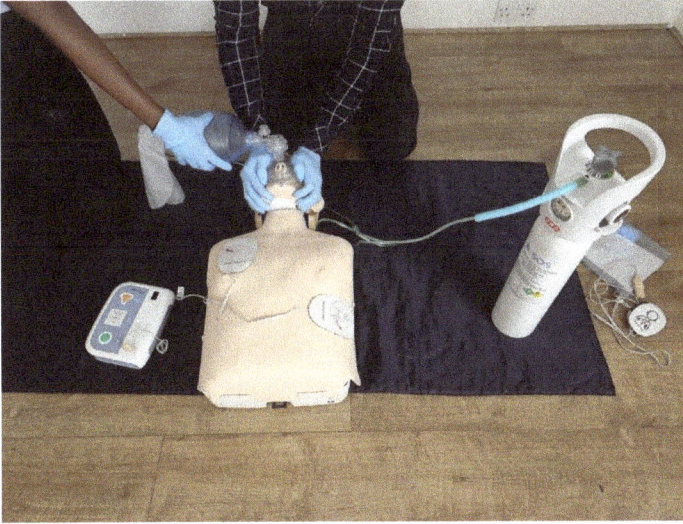

5) Use an AED (Automated External Defibrillator)

1. **Turn on the AED as soon as available**
2. **Attach pads** to the bare chest as shown on the pads
   - One pad on the **upper right chest**
   - One pad on the **left side below the armpit** (mid-axillary line)
3. Follow **voice prompts**.
4. **Deliver shock if advised**, then **resume CPR immediately**.
5. If three shocks fail, consider **changing pad position** (e.g., move the right-shoulder pad toward the centre of the chest to improve current flow) if trained.

6) Continue High-Quality CPR

- Continue CPR and AED cycles until:
  - **Signs of life return** (movement, normal breathing),
  - **Advanced responders take over**,
  - Or **you are unable to continue** due to exhaustion.

Special Considerations

If the arrest is due to drowning

→ Give **5 initial rescue breaths** before starting compressions, as hypoxia is the primary cause of arrest in these cases.

Vomiting or airway obstruction

✓ Ensure airway is clear
✓ Continue CPR with breaths if trained

SPECIAL SITUATION: CPR IN LATE PREGNANCY

When performing CPR on a heavily pregnant woman, raise the right hip slightly so that the pregnant woman is leaning slightly to the left side. This shifts the uterus away from the blood vessel, providing an uninterrupted blood supply to the heart.

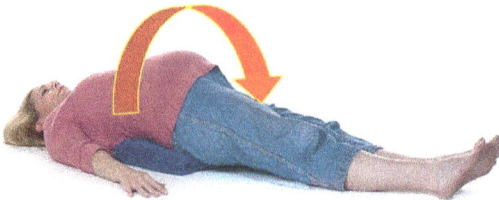

PREGNANT WOMEN & CPR

Unconscious and Breathing place her on her left side
(Labour Left)

CPR in a **pregnant woman** should be done in cycles of 30 compressions **and** two breaths. It is also safe to use an automated external defibrillator, or AED, if one is available.

CHILD CPR

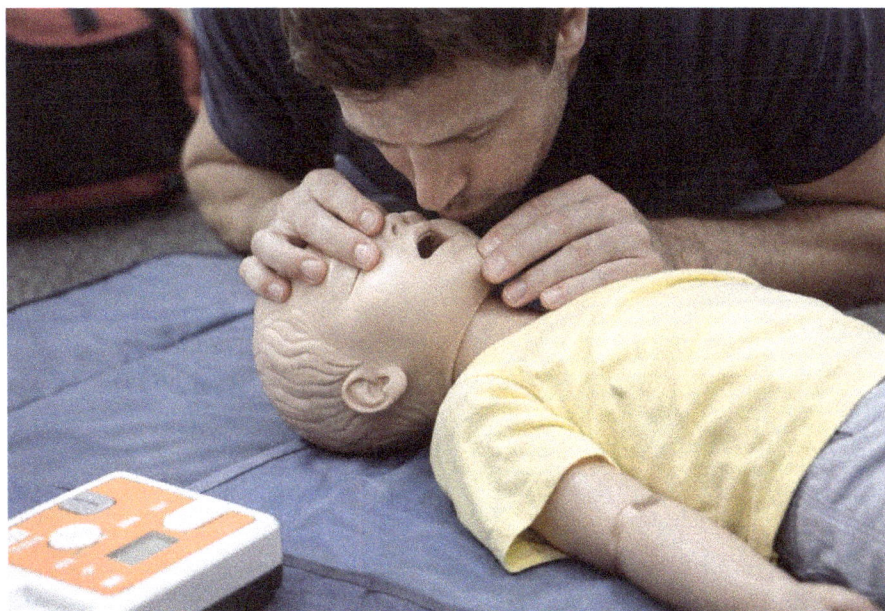

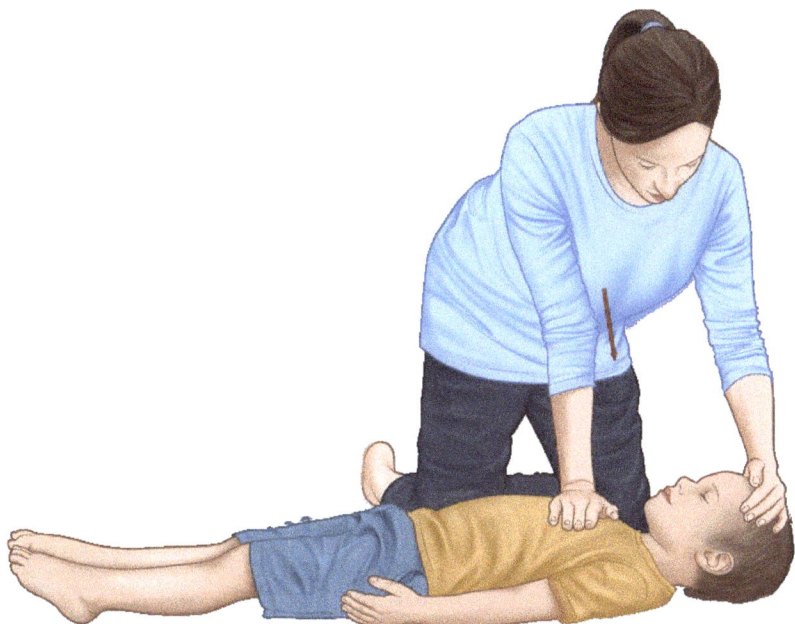

Key Differences

- Cardiac arrest is often **hypoxic**
- Rescue breaths are critical

Sequence

1. Danger
2. Response
3. Airway
4. Breathing
5. **5 initial rescue breaths**

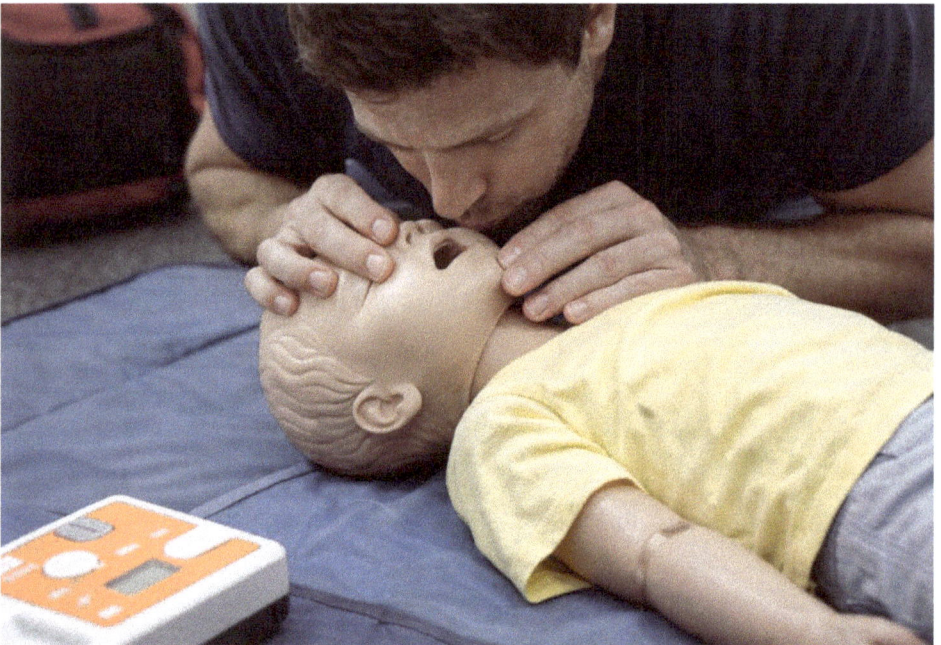

Chest Compressions

- One hand (or two for a larger child)

- Centre of chest
- Depth: ⅓ **of chest**
- Rate: **100–120 per minute**

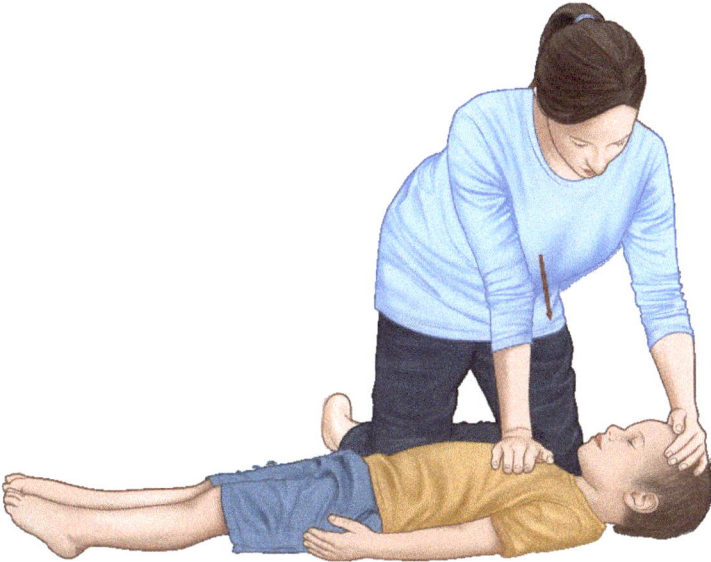

Compression–Ventilation Ratios

- **Healthcare professionals with paediatric duty: 15 compressions: 2 breaths**
- **Bystanders & most clinicians: 30 compressions: 2 breaths**

Defibrillation

- Use an AED immediately
- Use **paediatric pads** if available
- If pads touch → **front-and-back placement**

INFANT CPR (<1 year)

Response

- Tickle feet
- Observe for movement or sound

Call 999 or 112

Airway

- Neutral head position
- **One finger** chin lift only

Breathing

Give **five rescue breaths**

- Mouth-to-mouth

  Rescue breaths may be delivered using mouth-to-mouth-and-nose or via a bag-valve-mask, ensuring an effective seal.

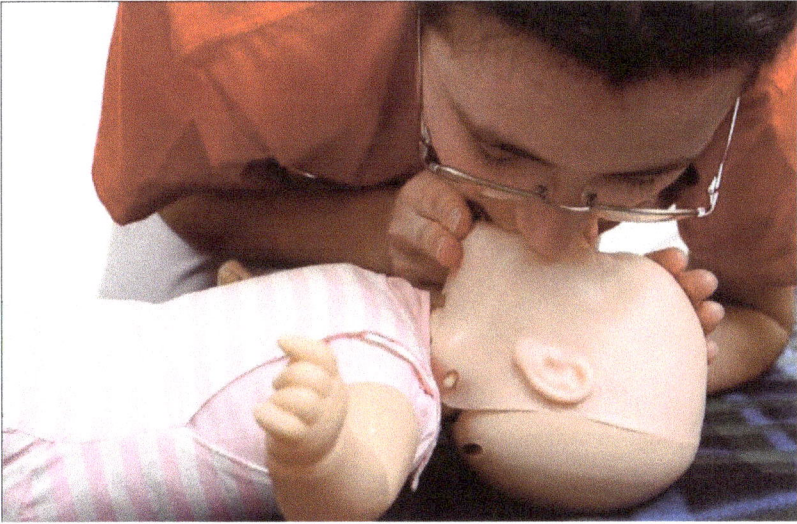

- Or mouth-to-nose if mouth injured

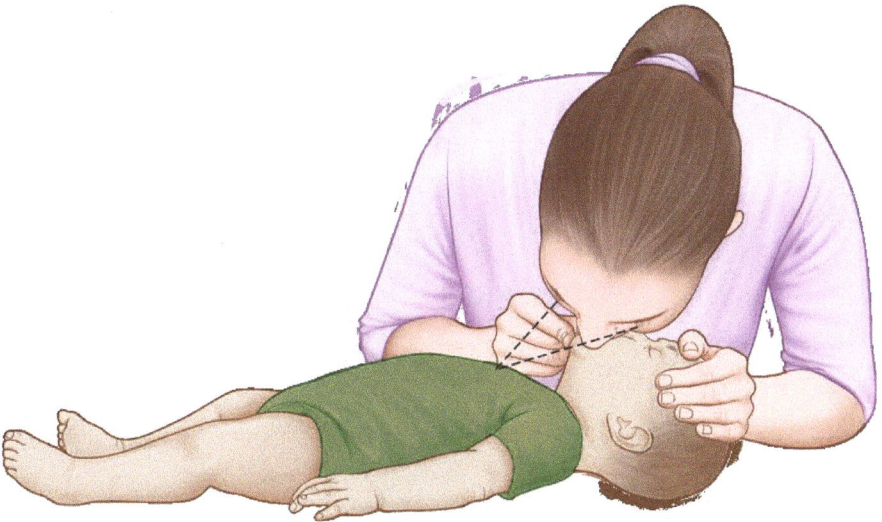

- Mouth to bag valve mask

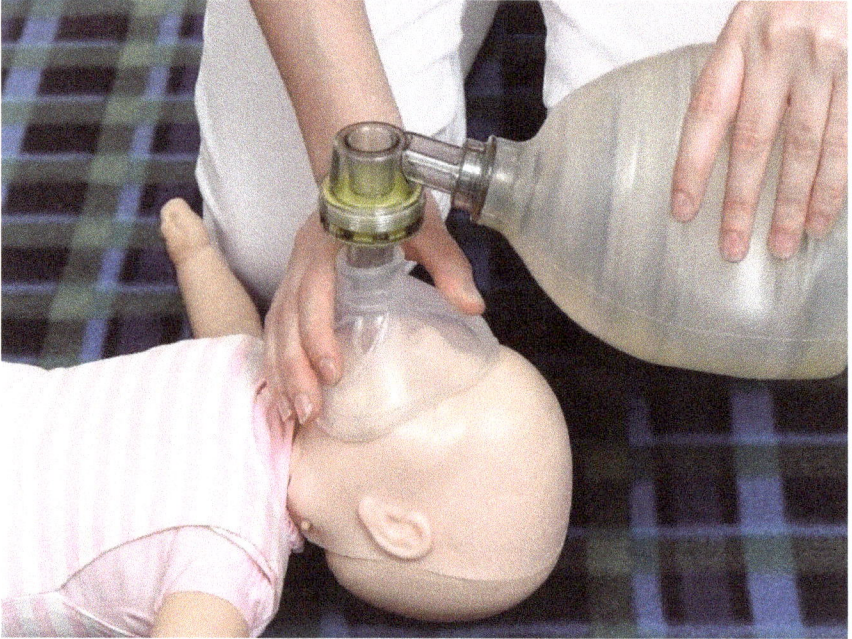

Chest Compressions

- Depth: ⅓ **of chest**

Ratios

- **Healthcare professionals with paediatric duty: 15:2**
- **Bystanders: 30:2**

Defibrillation

- Use an AED as soon as available
- Use paediatric pads if possible
- Pad placement: **front and back**

- Infant compressions with two thumbs

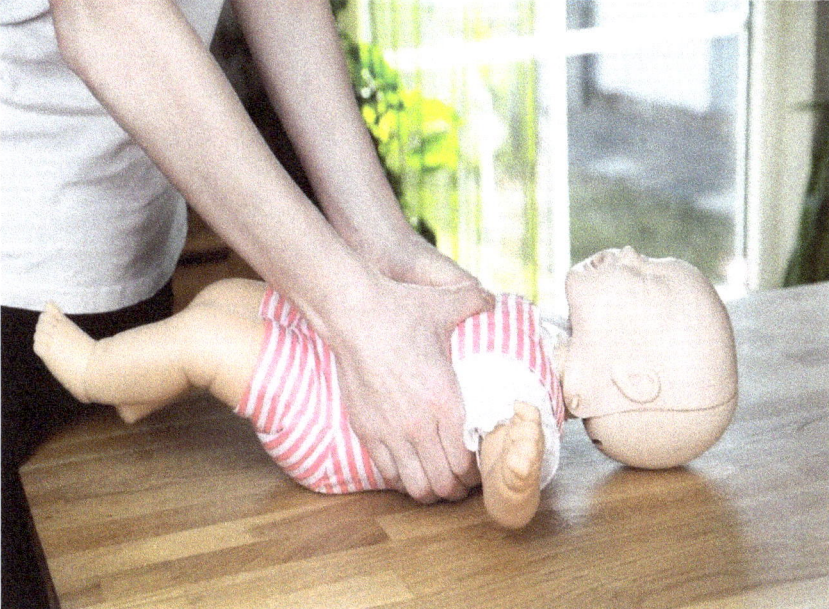

Fig 3. **Chest compression in infants: two-thumb encircling technique**

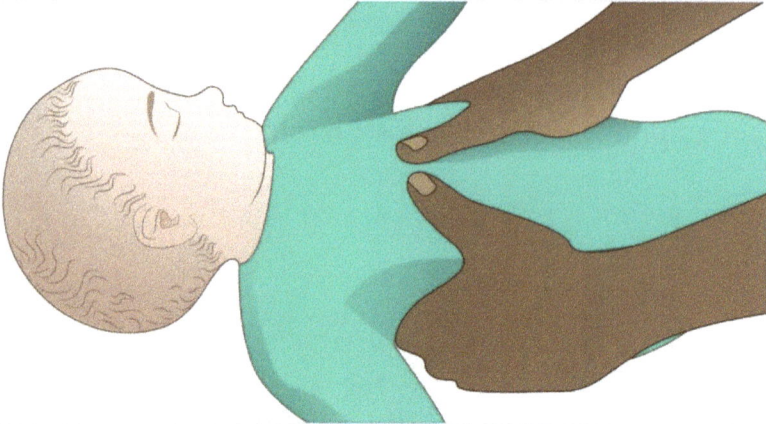

The two-thumb circling technique should be done with the thumbs side by side, and the hands encircling the infant's rib cage

DEFIBRILLATION

Key determinants of successful defibrillation:

- **Time to shock** – earlier defibrillation increases success
- **High-quality CPR** – before and between shocks maintains myocardial perfusion
- **Shockable rhythm** – VF and pulseless VT only
- **Myocardial condition** – oxygenation, perfusion, pH, and electrolytes
- **Correct energy & biphasic waveform**
- **Good pad position & contact** – low transthoracic impedance
- **Underlying cause** – primary cardiac causes respond best

DEFIBRILLATOR SIGNAGE

AED provision should follow national guidance, local policy, and risk assessment. All staff must know how to access and use an AED when available. The defibrillator signage must be properly displayed and visible to all members of staff and visitors to the healthcare environment..

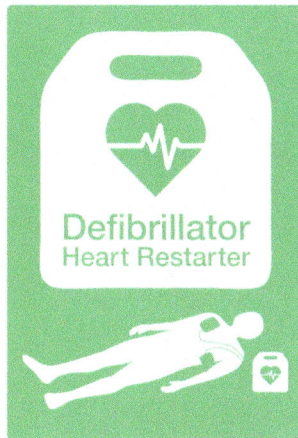

WHAT TO DO WHEN THE AED ARRIVES

Turn the machine on by pushing the on button. For most AEDs, the button will be green.

Making sure the casualty is bare-chested must be the case for all casualties, whether male or female, adult, or child. For female casualties, remove any bra and, if necessary, use scissors to cut through it.

Remove the electrodes or PADS from their seal and remove the backing paper to reveal the sticky part of the pads.

A defibrillator is a device that sends an electric shock to the heart to restore a normal heartbeat.

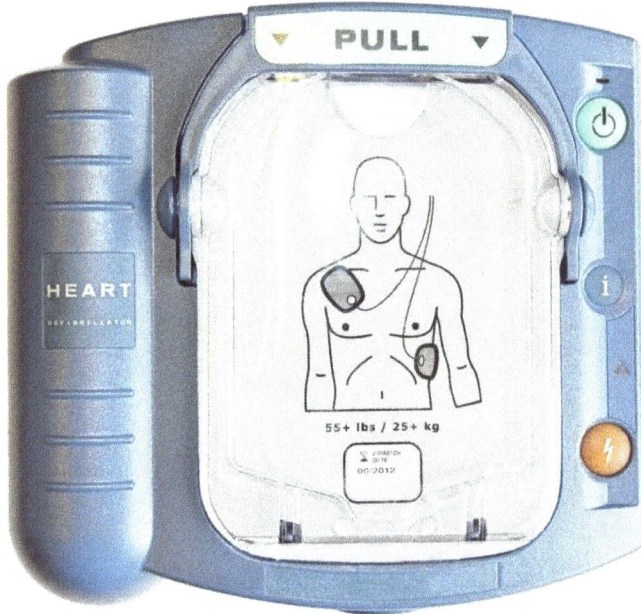

Steps for Using the AED

- When the AED arrives, turn the start button on, and it will automatically begin to issue instructions.

- Attach the electrode pads to the patient's bare chest.

- The AED will begin analysing the patient's heart rhythm. Do not touch the patient while the heart rhythm is being explored.

- If you have a semi-automatic defibrillator, it will ask you to press the shock button to deliver a shock if it detects a shockable rhythm.

Aftershock is delivered, and the AED will instruct you to continue CPR.

Common types of automated external defibrillators.

DEFIBRILLATOR SIGNAGE

Every dental practice must have a defibrillator, and staff must know where it is located. The defibrillator signage must be displayed appropriately and be visible to all staff and visitors to the practice.

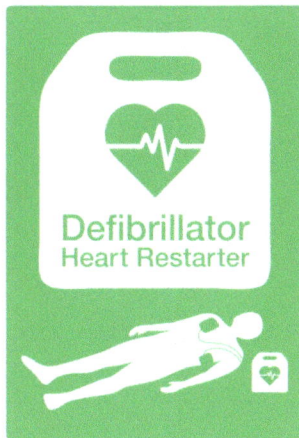

ATTACHING THE PADS

ANTERO-LATERAL PAD PLACEMENT

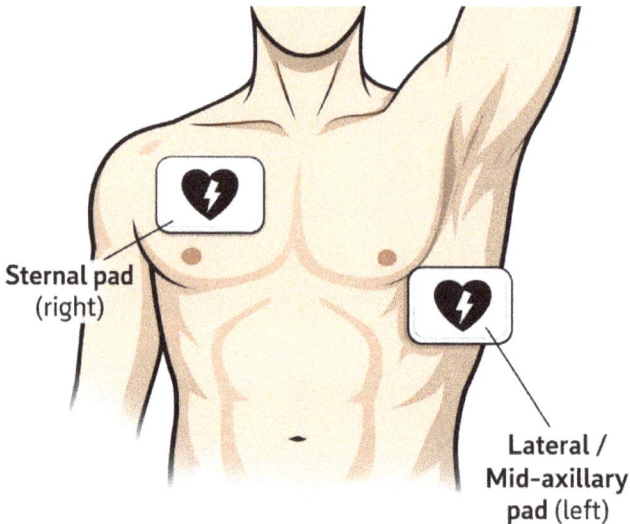

Sternal pad (right)

Lateral / Mid-axillary pad (left)

Adult AED Pad Placement (Anterior–Lateral)

Correct pad placement is essential to ensure effective defibrillation by allowing electrical current to pass through the myocardium.

Anterior (Sternal) Pad – Adult

- Place one pad on the **right upper chest**
- Position it **just below the right clavicle**
- Ensure it is **to the right of the sternum**

Lateral (Apical) Pad – Adult

- Place the second pad on the **left side of the chest**
- Position it **below the left armpit (axilla)**
- Align it with the **mid-axillary line**, level with the lower edge of the pectoral muscle (over the cardiac apex)

Rationale for Anterior–Lateral Pad Placement

This pad configuration:

- Allows the defibrillation current to pass **diagonally through the heart**
- Maximises the likelihood of successful defibrillation
- Prevents pad overlap
- Keeps pads clear of excessive breast tissue, muscle mass, and implanted devices (where possible)

Pads should always be applied **exactly as shown on the AED diagrams** when available.[29]

Key Clinical Points for Practice

- Remove excessive chest hair if pads will not adhere
- Ensure the chest is dry before pad application
- Do not delay defibrillation for pad repositioning unless placement is clearly incorrect
- Continue CPR immediately after shock delivery or if no shock is advised

References

29. Resuscitation Council UK. *Defibrillation and Automated External Defibrillators (AEDs) – Adult Basic Life Support*
30. European Resuscitation Council. *Guidelines for Resuscitation: Defibrillation*

Anteroposterior (AP) AED Pad Placement – Anterior Pad (Adult)

Anterior (Front) Pad

- Place the pad on the **left side of the chest**, over the **precordial area**
- Position it **to the left of the sternum**, overlying the heart
- **Do not place directly over the centre of the chest (sternum)**

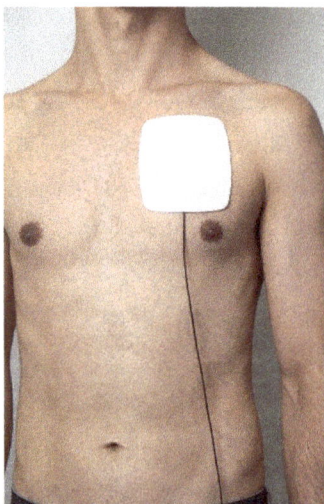

BACK(POSTERIOR) PAD

- Place the pad on the left side of the back
- Put it just below the left shoulder blade
- This pad is behind the heart

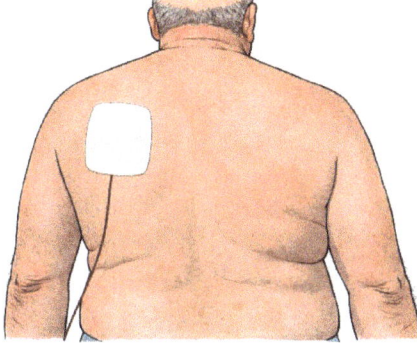

CHILD CPR- DEFIBRILLATING A CHILD- FRONT AND BACK PAD PLACEMENT.

1-12 years Front-Back

- Place the pads in the centre of the chest
- Position it between the nipples
- Back (posterior) pad
- Place on the centre of the back
- Position it between the shoulder blades

The goal is to have one pad on the chest and one on the back, with the heart between them.

CHILD 13-18 YEARS –

(ADOLESCENT) SAME AS ADULT

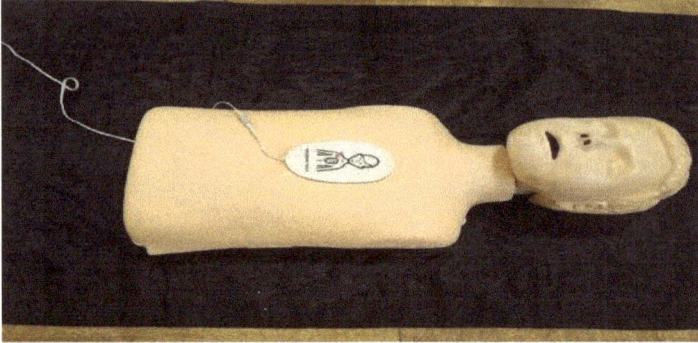

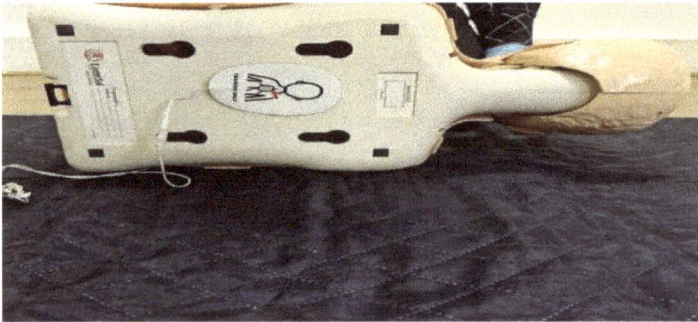

One pad on the upper right chest, and the other on the left side of the chest under the armpit.

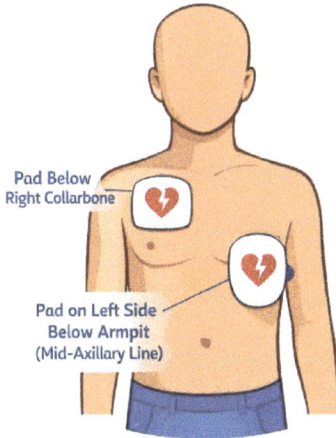

AED Pad Placement for Teen

Pad Below Right Collarbone

Pad on Left Side Below Armpit (Mid-Axillary Line)

HOW THE AED WORKS

- The pads have sensors called electrodes. When attached to the patient's chest, it sends information about the patient's heart rhythm to the AED's computer. The computer analyses the heart's rhythm to confirm whether a shock is necessary and, if required, will send a shock to correct the abnormal heart rhythm

TYPES OF DEFIBRILLATORS

- Automated External Defibrillators (AEDs)
- Implantable Cardioverter Defibrillators (ICDs)- surgically placed inside the body.

- Wearable Cardioverter Defibrillators (WCDs)-this rests on the body

SAFETY CONSIDERATIONS

JEWELLERY- remove pieces of jewellery and avoid placing the pads on them

MEDICATIONS- Do not place the pads on the pacemaker.

CLOTHING- The patient must be bare-chested.

WATER/SWEAT-wipe any water

MEDICATIONS do not place pads on the GTN patch.

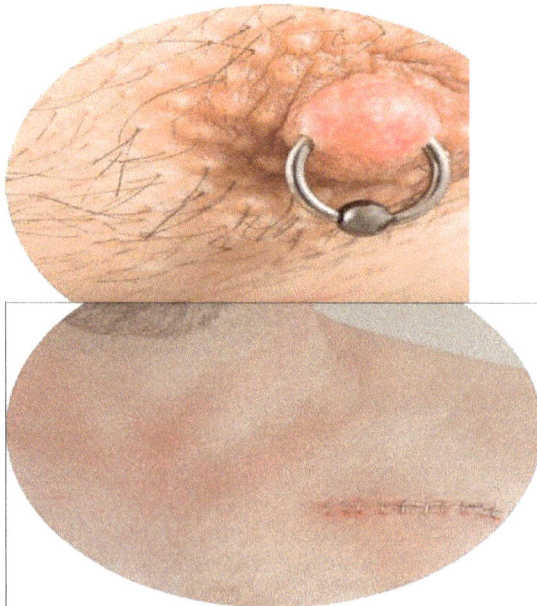

RESCUE BREATH METHODS (All Ages)

- Mouth-to-mouth
- Mouth-to-mask (preferred)
- Bag-Valve-Mask (BVM)
  - One-person: **C-E grip**
  - Two-person: One seals the mask, one squeezes the bag
- Mouth-to-nose (facial trauma)
- Mouth-to-stoma or tracheostomy (ventilate directly via stoma)

WHEN TO USE 15:2 IN CHILDREN

15:2

- Paediatric doctors & nurses
- Paramedics
- Emergency department staff

30:2

- Members of the public
- Dentists, GPs, school nurses
- Lone responders

Rationale: Simplicity and likelihood of adult CPR scenarios

RECOVERY POSITION (Breathing but Unresponsive adult)

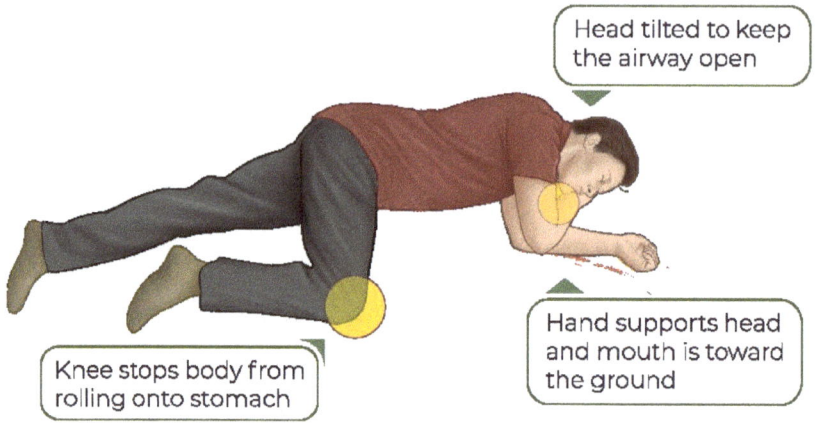

Head tilted to keep the airway open

Hand supports head and mouth is toward the ground

Knee stops body from rolling onto stomach

- Place in **lateral position**
- Head tilted, airway open
- Monitor breathing continuously

CHILD RECOVERY POSITION

CHECK FOR DANGER

Make sure you and the patient are safe.

CHECK FOR RESPONSIVENESS

Check whether the patient responds to a painful stimulus by squeezing the earlobes.

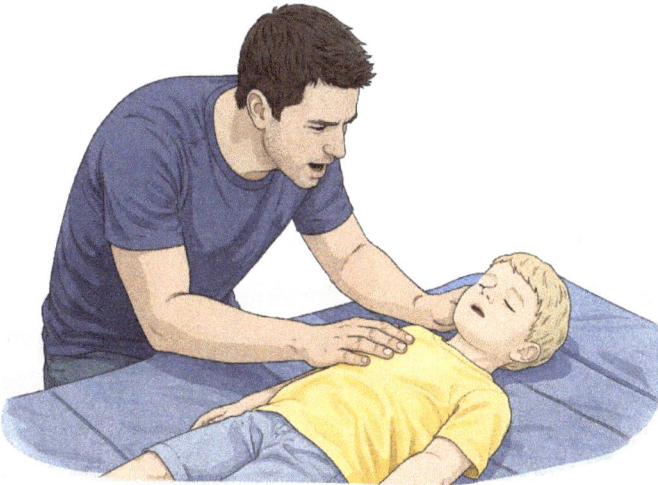

CHILD HEAD TILT, CHIN LIFT

Place one hand on the forehead and two fingers on the chin, tilt your head, and lift your chin.

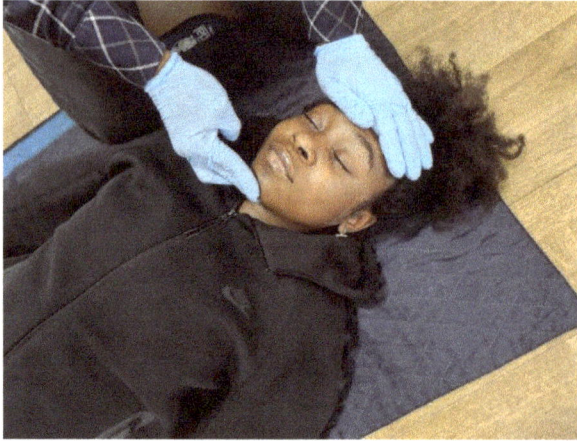

CHECK IF THE CHILD IS BREATHING

Lean towards the head with your cheek facing the casualty's nose to feel for the child's breath.

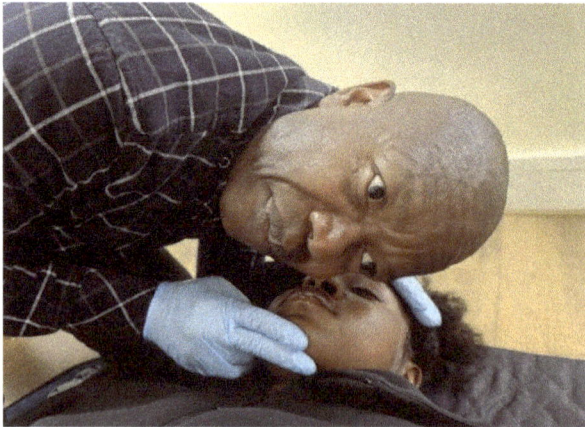

Reach for the casualty's hand nearest you and put it in an angled Or straight position.

Reach Out for The Casualty's Hand further from You. Place it On their Cheek And Hold It there.

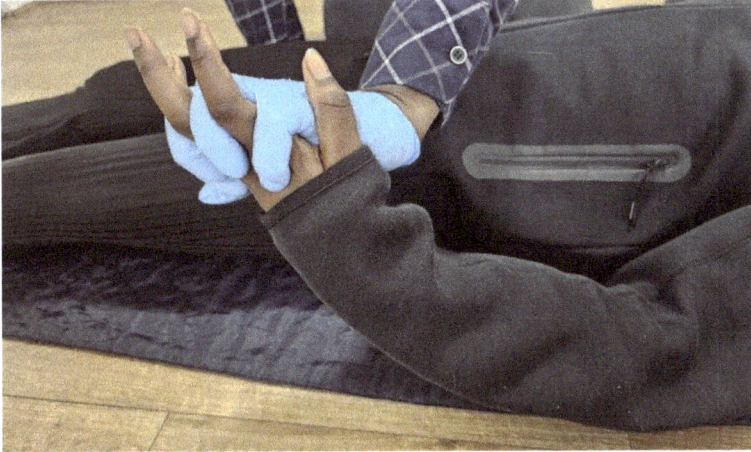

Place the back of the child's hand on their cheek and hold it palm to palm.

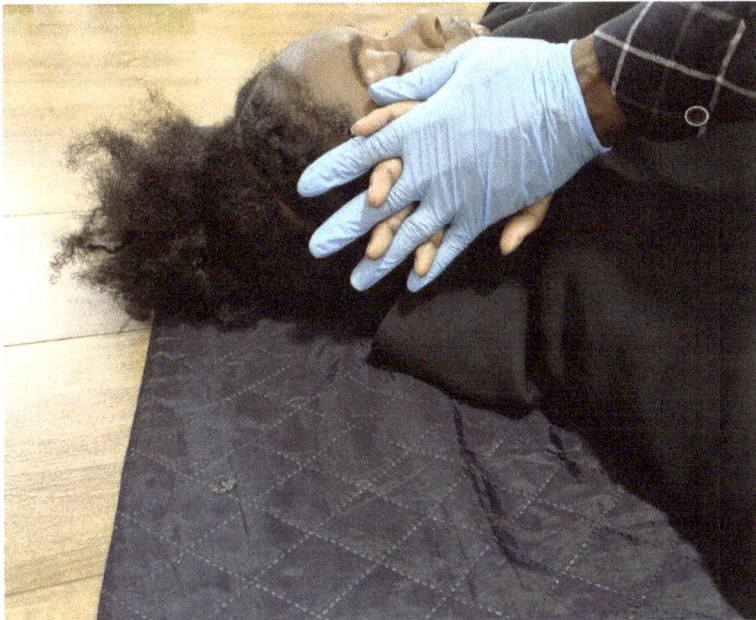

Check the pockets for any sharp objects likely to cause harm to the patient.

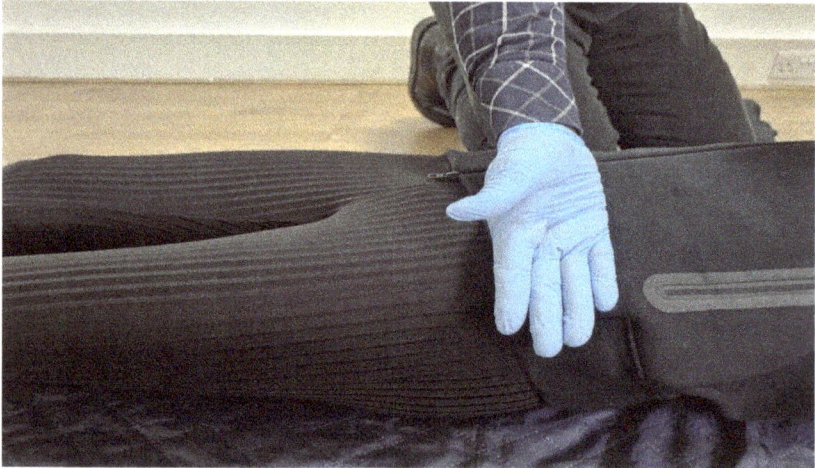

Check the pockets for Sharp objects that can harm the child when you are on her side.

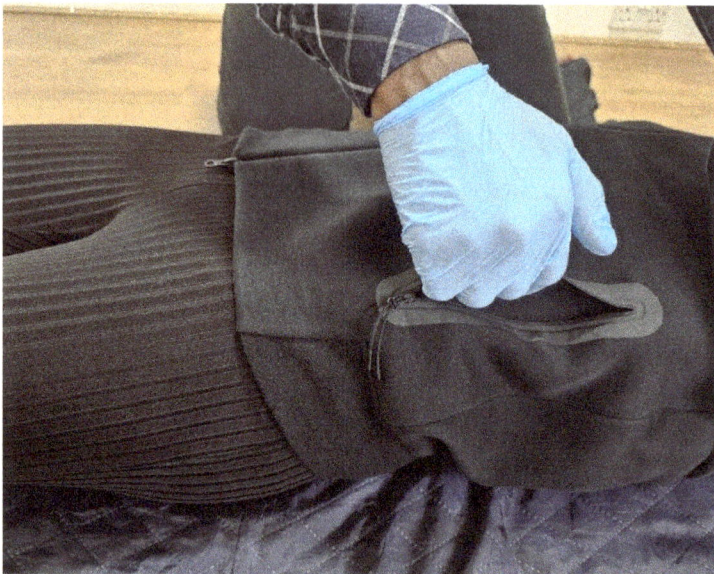

Place your hand on the outer part of the child's leg, which is furthest from you, around the knee.

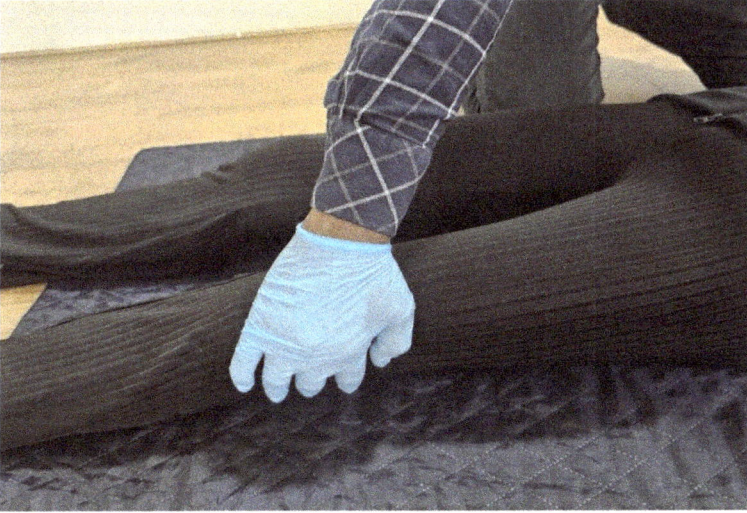

Reach for the leg farther from you and raise it from the Outer part of the knee area, Making Sure the feet are firmly on the ground. Then, lean the casualty towards you.

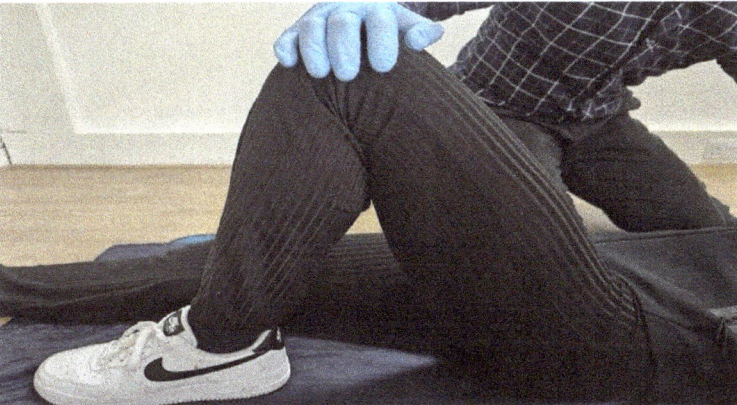

Lift the leg with your hand on the child's knee. Using the knee as a lever, roll the child on her side in a recovery position. Tilt the head back carefully to maintain a clear airway. Check every minute to confirm the child is still breathing whilst waiting for an ambulance to arrive.

TILT THE CHIN UP TO CLEAR THE CASUALTY'S AIRWAY

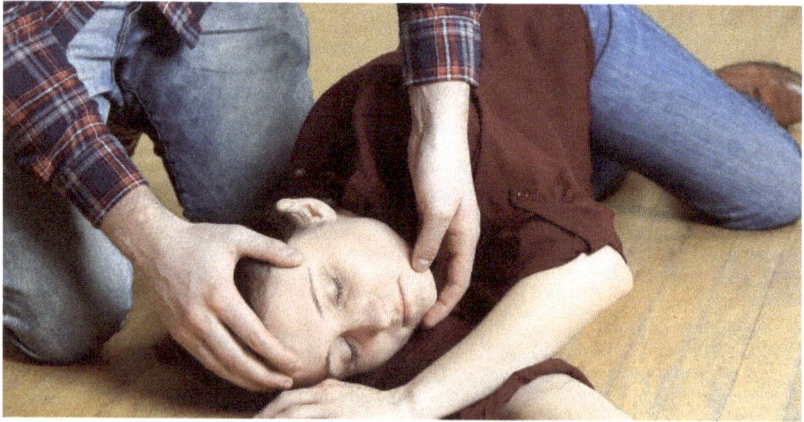

RECOVERY POSITION BABY

CHECK IF BABY IS RESPONSIVE

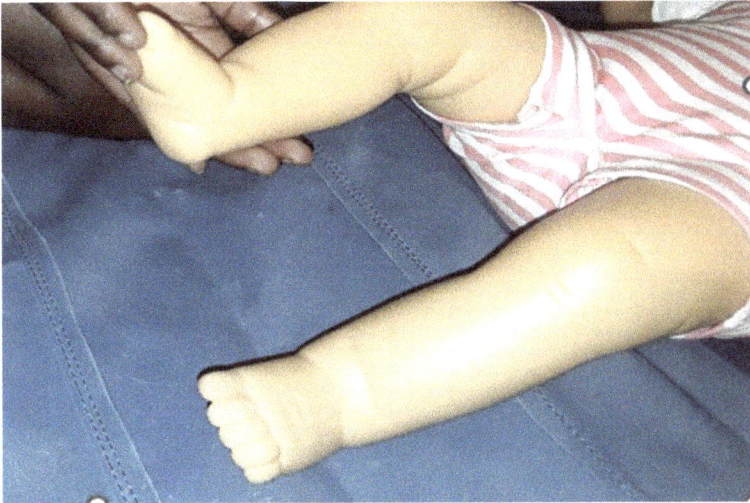

CALL 999/112 IF BABY IS UNRESPONSIVE

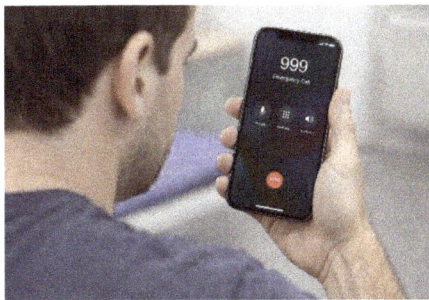

CHECK THE AIRWAY- HEAD TILT AND CHIN LIFT.

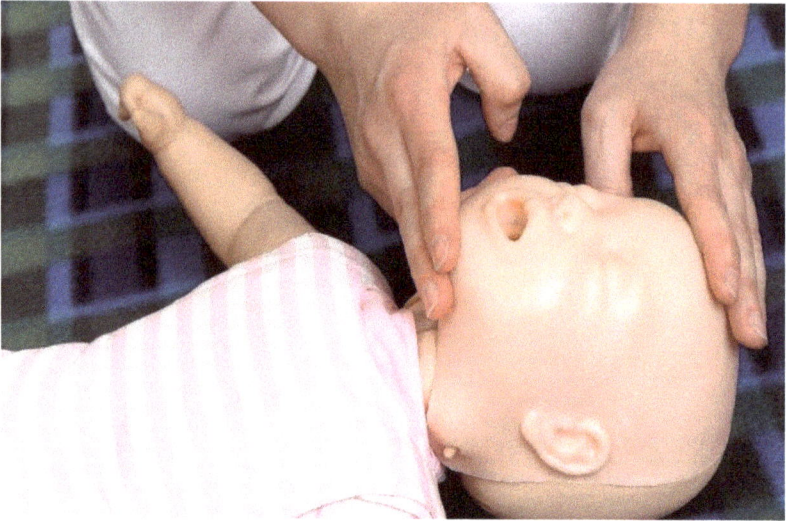

CHECK BREATHING.

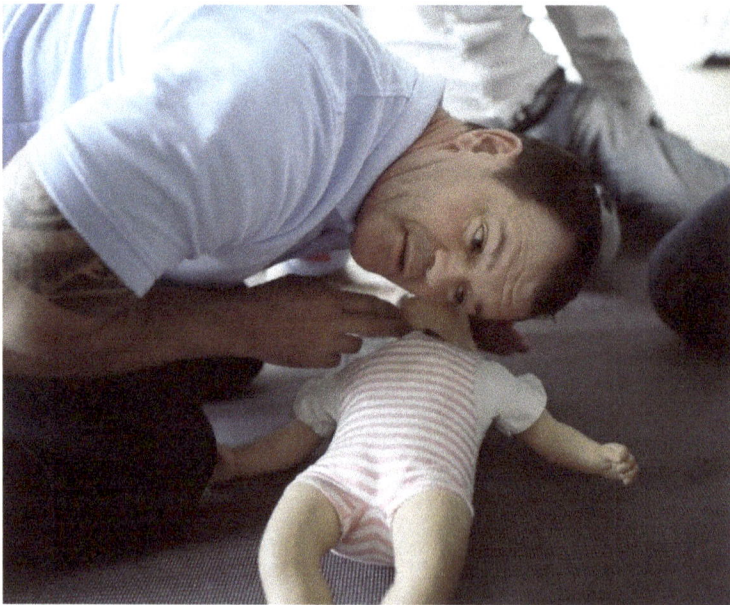

If an infant is unresponsive but breathing normally, maintain the airway in a neutral position, monitor continuously, and await emergency services.
If breathing becomes abnormal or stops, commence CPR immediately.

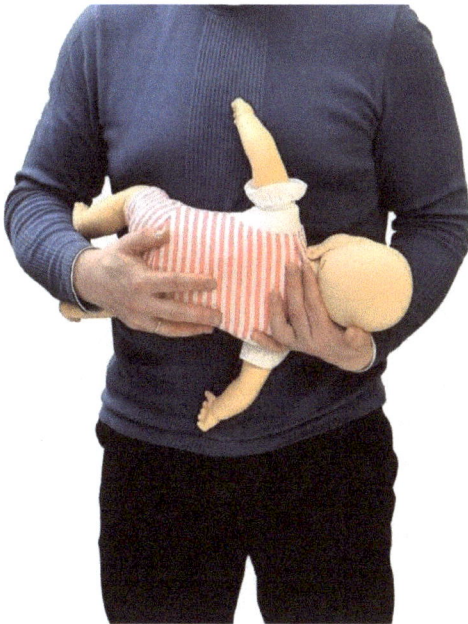

- Head lower than body
- Maintain airway alignment

ADULT CHOKING

WHAT IS CHOKING?

Choking occurs when the airway is partially or fully blocked, preventing air from reaching the lungs. This can happen anywhere from the mouth down to where the windpipe splits into the lungs.

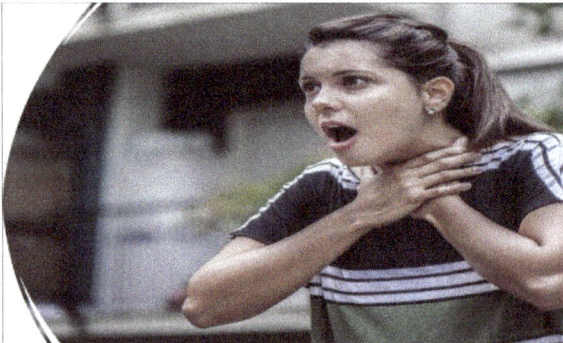

Mild Choking- adult

Mild choking occurs when the airway is only partially blocked, and the patient can still **breathe, cough, or speak**.

- **What to do:**
  - Encourage the patient to **cough forcefully**.
  - Do **not interfere** if they can clear the obstruction themselves.
  - **Do not give back blows or chest thrusts** unless the airway becomes entirely blocked.

Severe Choking

Severe choking usually involves complete blockage of the airway. The person will not be able to speak. To help them, you must immediately commence five back lows followed by five abdominal thrusts. If the treatment does not work, the patient will, at some point, become unconscious and not breathing. It would be best if you commenced CPR immediately.

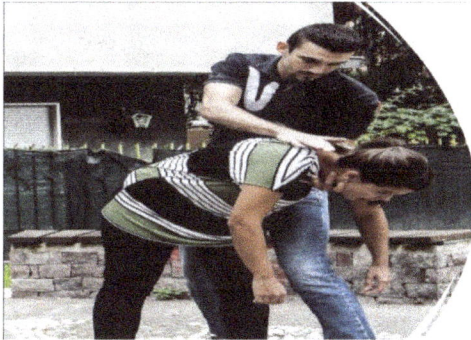

Abdominal thrusts

Make a fist with your dominant hand, and then place that fist above the navel and below the tip of the sternum. Press backward and upwards up to five times.

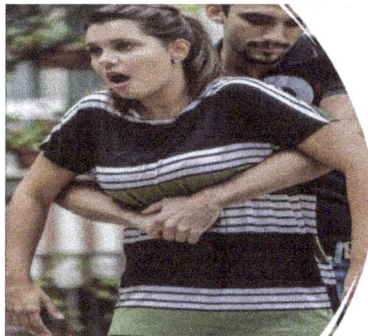

COMMON CAUSES IN PATIENTS

- Eating too quickly
- Loose or poorly fitting dentures
- Eating while lying down
- Not chewing properly
- Small objects, toys, or teeth
- Vomit

Signs of a child choking

- Suspect a foreign-body airway obstruction if a child or adolescent cannot speak, breathe, or cough effectively.
- **Call 999 or 112**
- Call **for help** if the obstruction persists or the patient shows signs of severe choking.

EMERGENCY ACTIONS FOR INFANTS (<1 YEAR)

SIGNS OF A CHOKING INFANT

How to help a choking child

Follow these steps if the child is choking:

1. CALL 999 FOR AN AMBULANCE

Ask for an ambulance and tell them the child is choking

My child is choking!

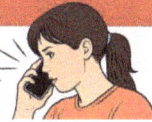

THEN

1. Give up to 5 back blows

Lean the child forward

Give 5 sharp back blows between the shoulder blades

Check if the choking is relieved after each blow

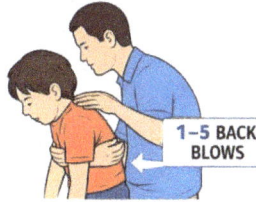

1–5 BACK BLOWS

2. Give up to 5 back blows:

If still choking, give abdominal thrusts:

Stand behind the child

Place your fist in the middle of the abdomen

Pull inwards and upwards up to 5 times

Check if the choking is relieved after each thrust

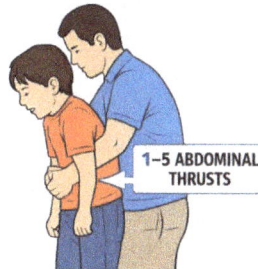

1–5 ABDOMINAL THRUSTS

✓ Continue with 5 back blows and 5 abdominal thrusts

✓ Follow the call handler's advice until help arrives

- Suspect choking when an infant has an ineffective cough, is unable to cry or vocalise, has cyanosis, or shows silent attempts to breathe

- **CALL FOR 999 OR 112**

- Call or have someone call the ambulance service as soon as possible.

GIVE 5 BACK BLOWS

Position the infant face down along your forearm, resting your arm on your thigh. Support the head and keep it lower than the chest. Deliver up to five sharp back blows between the shoulder blades, checking after each blow to see if the obstruction has cleared.

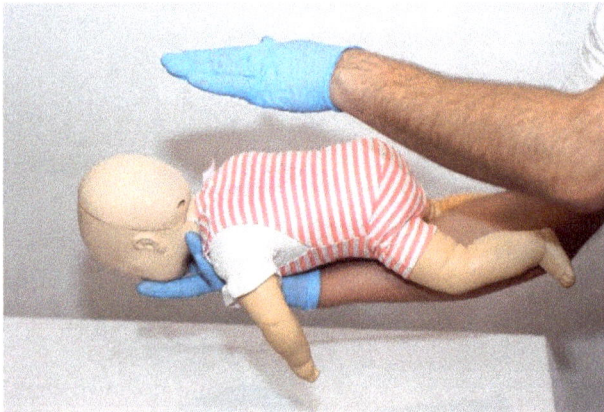

Chest Thrust with two thumbs encircling technique

Place the baby on their back on your lap. Wrap your hands around their chest and use your thumbs to give up to five quick pushes on the middle of the chest. Check after each push to see if the object has come out.

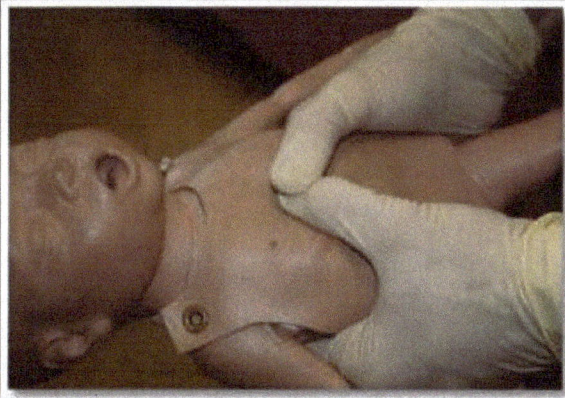

NO BLIND FINGER SWEEPS

Do not put your fingers blindly into the baby's mouth. Remove the object only if you can see it clearly.

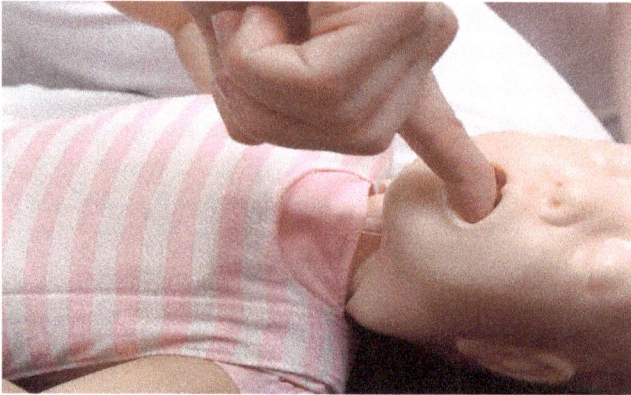

Do not put your fingers blindly into the baby's mouth. Remove the object only if you can see it clearly.

RESUSCITATION COUNCIL GUIDELINES ON THE USE OF SUCTION-BASED AIRWAY CLEARANCE DEVICES, SUCH AS LIFEVAC, FOR INDIVIDUALS IN HEALTHCARE ENVIRONMENTS.

The Resuscitation Council does not yet support the use of these devices because:

a. There are insufficient evidence and research on the safety of these anti-choking devices.
b. There is no evidence that they are effective.

c. The use of the devices may delay the use of established treatments for choking.

d. Trained healthcare professionals already use advanced techniques such as suction, laryngoscopes, and forceps to remove foreign bodies stuck in the airway.

OXYGEN

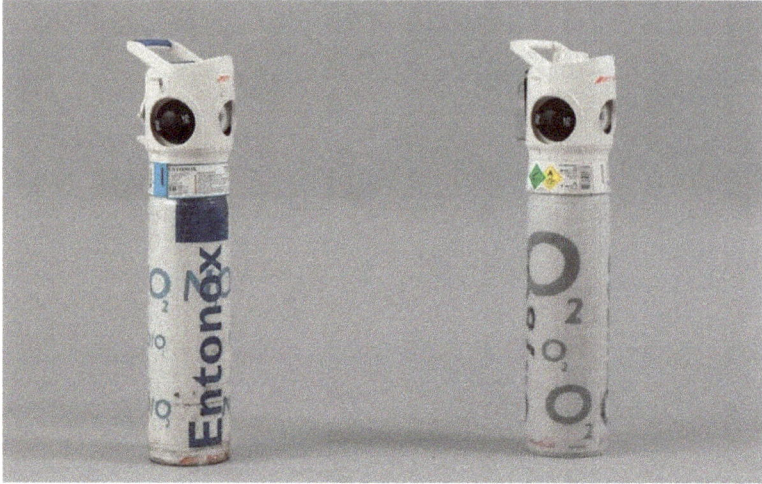

Oxygen Therapy in the Clinical Environment

Oxygen is a commonly used emergency drug in healthcare settings and must be administered **safely, appropriately, and according to national guidance**. In dental and primary care environments, the main gases encountered are **medical oxygen** and **Entonox® (50% oxygen / 50% nitrous oxide)**, both supplied in compressed cylinders of varying sizes.[31]

Types of Medical Gases

Medical Oxygen

- A **prescription-only medicine** used to treat hypoxaemia
- Delivered via masks or airway devices at controlled flow rates

Entonox®

- A fixed mixture of **50% oxygen and 50% nitrous oxide**
- Used primarily for **analgesia**, not routine oxygen therapy
- Requires specific training and equipment

Oxygen Equipment: Components

An emergency oxygen kit should include:

- Medical-grade oxygen cylinder
- Regulator with flow meter
- Oxygen tubing
- Non-rebreather mask with reservoir bag
- Bag-valve-mask (BVM) with reservoir
- Therapy (simple) face mask
- Resuscitation mask

Cylinders should be stored securely and handled in accordance with local safety policies.[32]

Oxygen Equipment Assembly (Emergency Use)

1. Place the oxygen cylinder securely (upright or safely supported)
2. Attach the **regulator** firmly to the cylinder
3. Connect oxygen tubing to the selected delivery device (mask or BVM)
4. Turn the cylinder **on slowly**
5. Set the flow rate according to clinical need

Flow Rate in Critical Illness

- **15 litres per minute (L/min)** via:

- o Non-rebreather mask
- o Bag-valve-mask with reservoir

6. Apply the mask securely over the patient's mouth and nose
7. Continuously monitor the patient's response and vital signs[33]

Discontinuing Oxygen Therapy

- Remove the oxygen mask when clinically appropriate
- Turn off the cylinder valve
- Allow the pressure gauge to fall to zero
- Disconnect equipment and replace the cylinder if empty

Record oxygen use in the patient chart.

Oxygen Delivery Devices

Non-Rebreather Mask

- Delivers **high-concentration oxygen**
- Flow rate: **10–15 L/min**
- Includes a reservoir bag and one-way valves to prevent re-breathing[33]

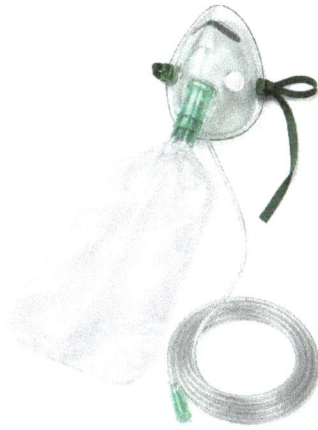

Simple Face Mask

- Has side ports allowing entrainment of room air
- Delivers **moderate oxygen concentrations**
- Requires flow rates ≥ 5 L/min to prevent CO_2 rebreathing

Venturi Mask

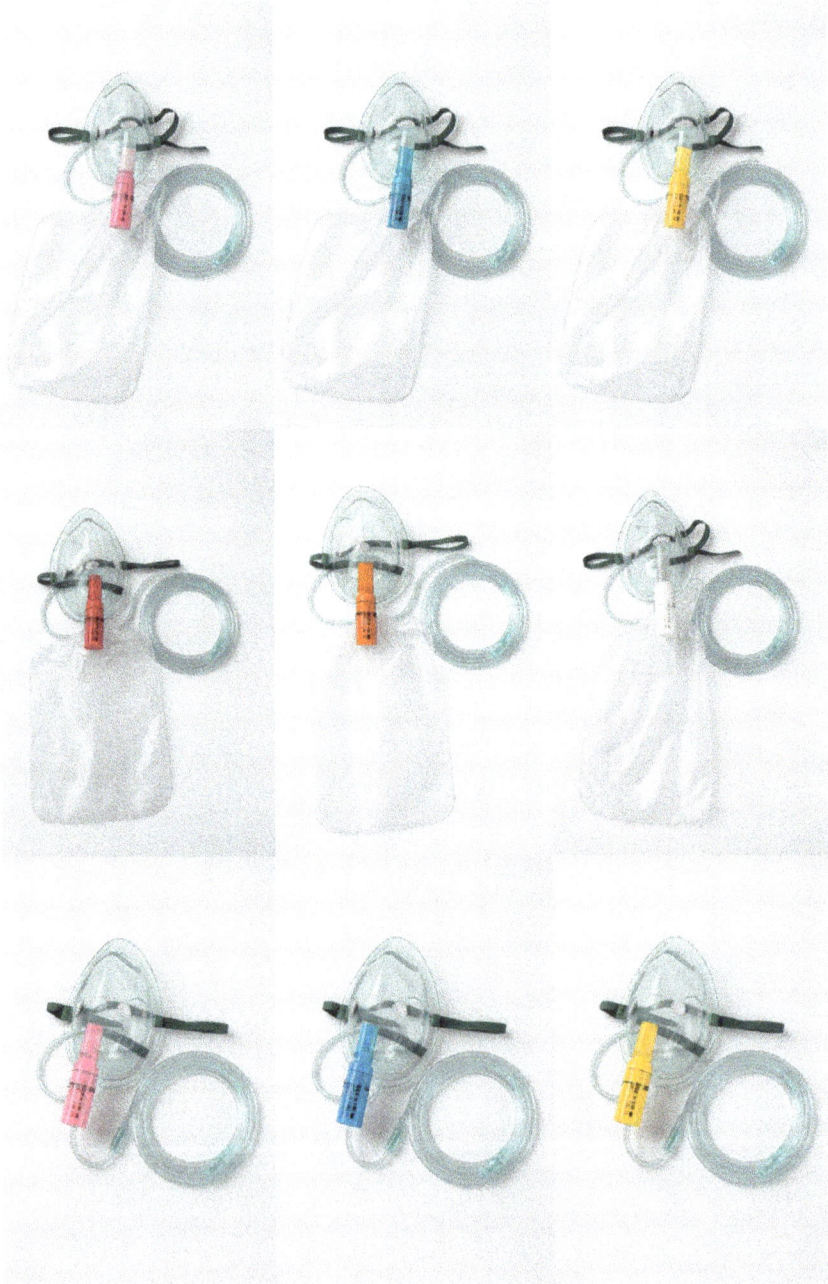

- Uses colour-coded valves to deliver **fixed oxygen concentrations**
- Particularly useful for patients at risk of **hypercapnic respiratory failure** (e.g. COPD)[34]

Nasal Cannula

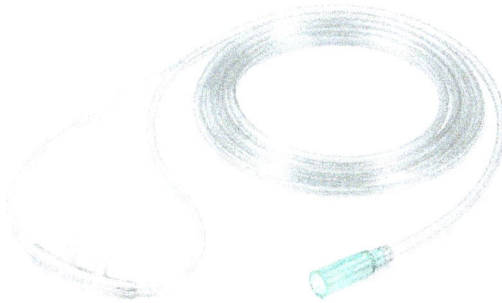

- Delivers low-flow oxygen via nasal prongs
- Flow rate: **1–4 L/min**
- Suitable for stable patients with mild hypoxia

Nebuliser

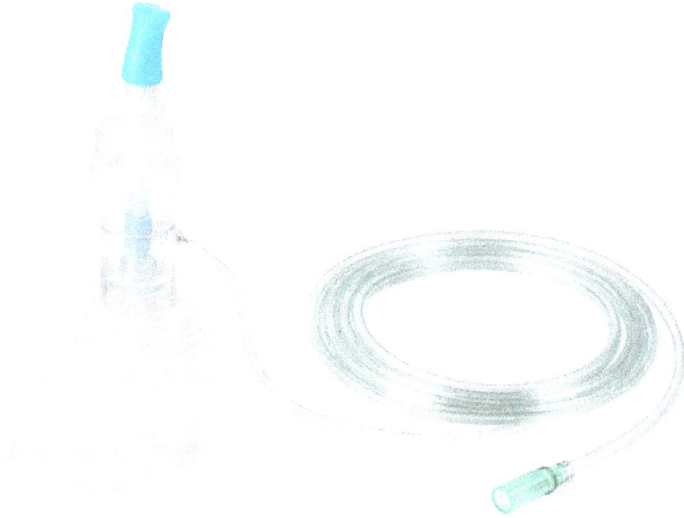

- Used to deliver **aerosolised medications**, not oxygen alone
- Oxygen or air may be used as the driving gas depending on the indication

Oxygen: Clinical Classification

- **Drug class:** Medical gas
- **Action:** Increases oxygen availability for cellular metabolism
- **Indications include:**
    - Hypoxaemia
    - Cardiac arrest
    - Shock
    - Severe asthma
    - Anaphylaxis

- o Carbon monoxide poisoning
- o Major trauma[33]

Adverse Effects and Cautions

- Excessive oxygen may:
  - o Reduce respiratory drive in patients with **chronic CO$_2$ retention**
  - o Cause **hypercapnia** in susceptible individuals (e.g. COPD)
  - o Lead to coronary vasoconstriction in certain cardiac conditions[34]

Oxygen should be **titrated to target saturations**, not given indiscriminately except in life-threatening emergencies.

Contraindications

- **Paraquat poisoning**
  Oxygen may worsen lung injury and should be avoided unless specifically advised by toxicology services[35]

Oxygen Dosage Summary (Adults)

Delivery Method	Flow Rate
Nasal cannula	1–4 L/min
Simple face mask	≥5 L/min
Venturi mask	As per valve colour
Non-rebreather mask	10–15 L/min
BVM with reservoir	15 L/min

References

31. British Thoracic Society. *Guideline for Oxygen Use in Adults in Healthcare and Emergency Settings*

32. Health and Safety Executive. *Safe Use of Compressed Gas Cylinders*

33. Resuscitation Council UK. *Emergency Oxygen Use and Adult Basic Life Support*

34. NICE. *Chronic Obstructive Pulmonary Disease in Over 16s (NG115)*

35. TOXBASE / UK National Poisons Information Service. *Paraquat Poisoning*

ANAPHYLAXIS –
EMERGENCY MANAGEMENT ALGORITHM (UK)

RECOGNISE ANAPHYLAXIS

Sudden onset (minutes) of illness **PLUS** any of the following:

A Airway

✓ Throat tightness
✓ Hoarse voice
✓ Tongue / lip swelling
✓ Stridor

B Breathing

✓ Shortness of breath
✓ Wheeze / bronchospasm
✓ Rapid breathing
✓ Cyanosis

⚠ **Skin signs** (urticaria, flushing, angioedema) may be **ABSENT**

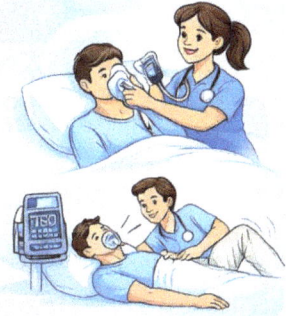

IMMEDIATE ACTIONS (ABCDE)

1. CALL FOR HELP

Activate emergency reponse
Call 999 / 112 or local resuscitation team

2. POSITION

✓ **Lie patient flat**
✓ If breathing severely
   compromised — semi-reclined
✓ Pregnancy: left lateral tilt

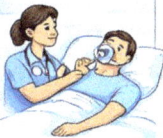

C Circulation

✓ Dizziness or collapse
✓ Hypotension
✓ Tachycardia
✓ Pale, clammy skin
✓ Loss of consciousness

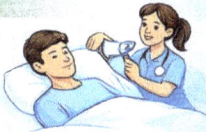

🔄 **Repeat every 5 minutes** if no improvement

5. AIRWAY & BREATHING

✓ **High-flow oxygen** (15 L/min)
✓ Monitor **SpO$_2$, RR**
✓ Prepare suction
✓ Anticipate airway obstruction

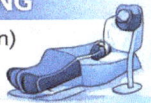

COMMON PITFALLS

☒ Delaying adrenaline
☒ Retying on skin signs
☒ Sitting hypotensive patiients upright
☒ Using antihistaminesor salbutamol instead of
   adrenaline

2. POSITION

✓ Lie patient flat
✓ If breathing severely
   compromised — semi-reclined
✓ Pregnancy: left lateral tilt

☒ **Do NOT** allow patient to **stand or sit
   upright** if hypotensive

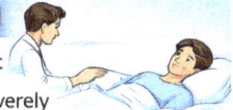

🔄 **Repeat every 5 minutes** if no improvement

4. AIRWAY & BREATHING
(AFTER ADRENALINE)

✓ **High-flow oxygen** (15 L/min)
✓ Monitor **SpO$_2$, RR**
✓ Prepare suction
✓ Anticipate airway obstruction

5. ONGOING CARE

✓ Continue ABCDE reassessment
✓ Prepare for **transfer** to hospital
✓ **Observe** for biphasic reaction
✓ Document: Trigger:
   Time of onset
✓ Drugs & doses
   Patient response

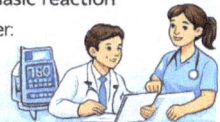

⚠ **KEY MESSAGE: *If in doubt —***
GIVE ADRENALINE

ANAPHYLAXIS – EMERGENCY MANAGEMENT ALGORITHM (UK)

Definitions: Allergic Reaction, Anaphylaxis, and Anaphylactic Shock

Allergic Reaction

An **allergic reaction** is a **mild to moderate immune response** to an allergen that **does not cause life-threatening compromise of the airway, breathing, or circulation**.

Features

- Localised urticaria or itching
- Mild angioedema
- Rhinitis or mild GI symptoms
- **Haemodynamically stable**

Management

- Antihistamines ± observation
- **Adrenaline not required**

Anaphylaxis

Anaphylaxis is a **severe, rapid-onset, life-threatening systemic hypersensitivity reaction** causing **airway, breathing, and/or circulation compromise**, often with skin or mucosal changes (which may be absent).

Features

- Throat tightness, hoarse voice, tongue swelling
- Wheeze, dyspnoea, hypoxia
- Hypotension, collapse, tachycardia

Management

- **Immediate IM adrenaline**
- ABCDE approach and emergency escalation

Anaphylactic Shock

Anaphylactic shock is the **most severe form of anaphylaxis**, characterised by **persistent hypotension and circulatory failure** leading to **inadequate tissue perfusion**.

Features

- Profound hypotension
- Collapse or reduced consciousness
- Pale, clammy skin, weak pulses

Management

- **Repeated adrenaline**
- High-flow oxygen, IV fluids
- Advanced resuscitation and critical care

Quick Comparison

Feature	Allergic Reaction	Anaphylaxis	Anaphylactic Shock
Life-threatening	No	Yes	Yes (critical)
ABC compromise	No	Yes	Severe
Hypotension	No	Possible	Persistent
Adrenaline required	No	**Yes**	**Yes (repeated)**

Key Message

If airway, breathing, or circulation are affected — treat as anaphylaxis and give adrenaline.

RECOGNISE ANAPHYLAXIS

Sudden onset (minutes) of illness PLUS any of the following:

Airway

- Throat tightness
- Hoarse voice
- Tongue/lip swelling
- Stridor

Breathing

- Shortness of breath

- Wheeze / bronchospasm
- Rapid breathing
- Cyanosis
- Falling SpO_2

Circulation

- Dizziness or collapse
- Hypotension
- Tachycardia
- Pale, clammy skin
- Loss of consciousness

Skin signs (urticaria, flushing, angioedema) may be ABSENT

IMMEDIATE ACTIONS (ABCDE)

1. CALL FOR HELP

- Activate emergency response
- Call **999 / 112** or the local resuscitation team

2. POSITION

- **Lie patient flat**
- If breathing is severely compromised → **semi-reclined**
- **Pregnancy:** left lateral tilt
- ✗ **Do NOT allow patient to stand or sit upright if hypotensive**

3. ADRENALINE (EPINEPHRINE) – FIRST LINE

DO NOT DELAY

Route

- **Intramuscular (IM)**

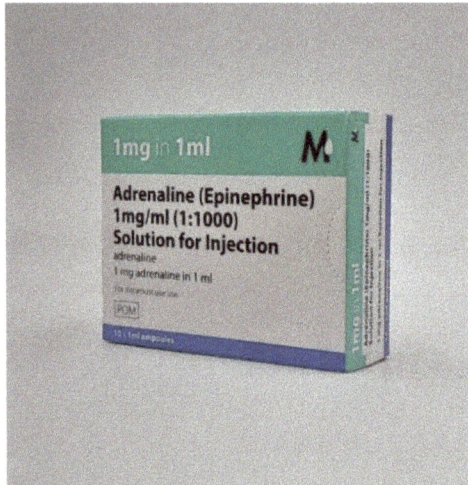

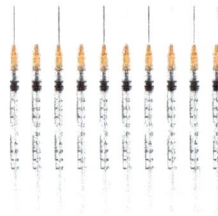

Site

- **Anterolateral thigh (vastus lateralis)**

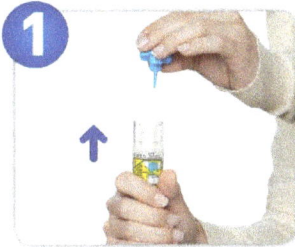

Form fist around EpiPen® and
BLUE SAFETY RELEASE

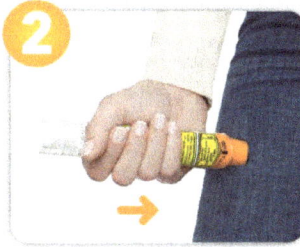

Push ORANGE end hard into outer
thigh so it 'clicks' and hold for 3 s‡

‡After administration of EpiPen® Adrenaline Auto-Injector
always seek medical attention – call **999 / 112**

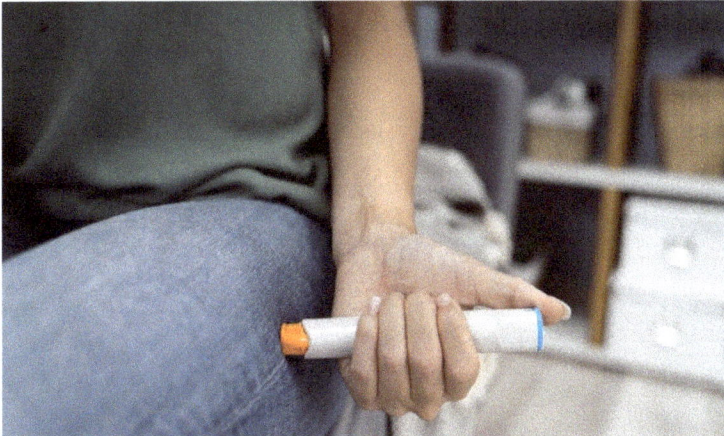

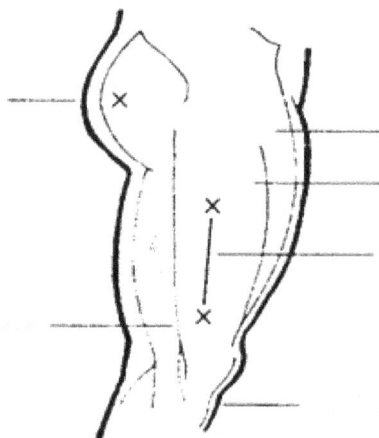

Dose (1:1000 = 1 mg/mL)

Patient	Dose
Adult	**500 micrograms (0.5 mL)**
Child 6–12 yrs	300 micrograms (0.3 mL)
Child 6 months–6 yrs	150 micrograms (0.15 mL)
Infant <6 months	100 micrograms (0.1 mL)

Repeat every 5 minutes if no improvement

IV adrenaline only by experienced clinicians in monitored settings

4. AIRWAY & BREATHING

- High-flow **oxygen (15 L/min)**
- Monitor **SpO₂, Respiratory rate.**

- Prepare suction
- Anticipate airway obstruction

5. CIRCULATION

- Monitor **pulse, BP, ECG**
- Gain **IV access**
- **IV fluids** for hypotension/shock (crystalloid bolus)

ADJUNCT TREATMENTS (AFTER ADRENALINE)

Must NOT delay adrenaline

- **Salbutamol** for persistent bronchospasm
- **Antihistamines** for persistent skin symptoms **only**
- **Corticosteroids NOT routine** in acute management

ONGOING CARE

- Continue **ABCDE reassessment**
- Prepare for **transfer to hospital**
- Observe for **biphasic reaction**
- Document:
  - Trigger
  - Time of onset
  - Drugs & doses
  - Patient response

COMMON PITFALLS

✗ Delaying adrenaline
✗ Relying on skin signs
✗ Sitting hypotensive patients upright
✗ Using antihistamines or salbutamol instead of adrenaline

KEY MESSAGE

If in doubt — GIVE ADRENALINE

NASAL ADRENALINE SPRAY FOR ANAPHYLAXIS

What is EURneffy®?

EURneffy® is a **needle-free adrenaline (epinephrine) nasal spray** used for the **emergency treatment of severe allergic reactions (anaphylaxis)**. It offers an alternative to traditional adrenaline auto-injectors (AAIs). [1]

---

[1] GOV.UK

Fast administration of adrenaline during anaphylaxis saves lives. A nasal spray may reduce hesitation to treat because it **avoids needles** and can be **used[2] quickly** in emergencies.

Regulatory Status

- GB **Approved by the UK's MHRA (July 2025)** — first needle-free option for anaphylaxis in the UK for adults and children ≥ 30 kg. Expected to be **available now (late 2025)**.
- EU **Approved by the European Commission (2024)** — authorised across EU Member States.

Who Can Use It?

Adults and **children weighing 30 kg or more** Prescription-only medicine — must be prescribed by a healthcare professional. [3]

How It Works (Quick Summary)

- A **single-use nasal spray** containing **2 mg adrenaline**.[4]
- Delivered **into one nostril only** — ready to use with no priming needed. (EURneffy®)
- Adrenaline is absorbed through the nasal lining and enters the bloodstream quickly to counteract anaphylaxis.[5]

---

[3] Anaphylaxis Campaign
[4] EURneffy®
[5] Anaphylaxis Campaign

When to Use It

Use EURneffy **as soon as signs of anaphylaxis appear**, such as:

- Difficulty breathing or wheeze
- Throat tightness or swelling
- Light-headedness/collapse
- Rapid onset of hives and low blood pressure

Administer immediately and call 999 — adrenaline is time-critical in anaphylaxis. [6]

Important Dosing & Administration Notes

✔ **One dose per device.** After use, the device must be discarded. [7]

✔ **Carry two devices** at all times — a second dose may be needed if symptoms continue or worsen. [8]
✔ **Seek urgent medical help after use**, even if symptoms improve[9]

Compared to Auto-Injectors

Advantages

- **Needle-free** — easier use for some patients
- **Smaller and lighter** to carry

---

[6] European Medicines Agency (EMA)
[7] EURneffy®
[8] (Anaphylaxis Campaign)

[9] European Medicines Agency (EMA)

- **Better temperature stability** and potentially longer shelf life than some auto-injectors [10]

Note: Traditional auto-injectors remain widely used and established; EURneffy is an additional option. Proper training in all adrenaline-delivery methods remains essential.

Safety & Side Effects

Common reported effects may include:

- Nasal discomfort or irritation
- Headache or congestion
- Throat irritation
- Nervousness, dizziness
  (*Common side effects seen with nasal adrenaline sprays in general — see full prescribing info for details.*) [11]

Key Learner Takeaways

- EURneffy is a **needle-free adrenaline spray** for emergency anaphylaxis treatment.
- Approved in the **UK and EU** for adults and children ≥ 30 kg.
- **Use immediately** on the first signs of anaphylaxis and **call emergency services**.
- Always **carry two devices**.

---

[10] (Pharma Focus Europe)

- Does **not replace emergency medical care** — hospital assessment is needed after use.

How to Use
EURneffy® Nasal Adrenaline Spray

Emergency treatment of severe allergic reaction (anaphylaxis)

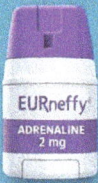

1. CALL 999 IMMEDIATELY

2. REMOVE SAFETY CAP — PULL OFF

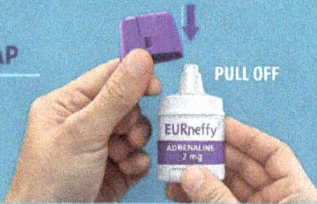

3. INSERT INTO 1 NOSTRIL

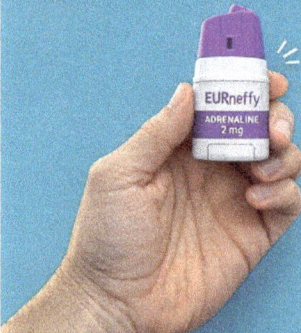

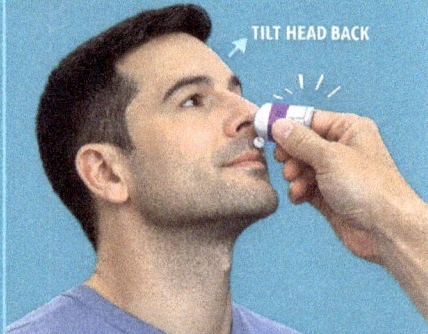

3. INSERT INTO 1 NOSTRIL — TILT HEAD BACK

USE ONE SPRAY ONLY | THEN SEEK MEDICAL HELP.

Use of Adrenaline Auto-Injectors Prescribed for a Named Patient

Is it permissible to administer an adrenaline auto-injector prescribed for one individual to a different patient?

No.
Under current UK medicines legislation, an **adrenaline auto-injector (AAI) that has been prescribed for a named individual may only be administered to that named person**.

Although **anyone may administer adrenaline to save a life in an emergency**, this legal exemption **does not extend to using a Prescription Only Medicine that has been specifically prescribed to someone else** when that medicine is an **adrenaline auto-injector**.

Legal Position

- **Adrenaline (epinephrine)** is a Prescription Only Medicine (POM).
- **Human Medicines Regulations 2012 (Regulation 238)** allow *any person* to administer a POM **by injection** in a life-threatening emergency **to save life**.
- However, this exemption **does not permit the use of a patient-specific prescribed medicine on another person** when that medicine is an **adrenaline auto-injector**.

Resuscitation Council (UK) Statement

"Currently, the law does not allow a non-prescriber to administer an adrenaline auto-injector which has been specifically prescribed for a named person to someone other than the person for whom it has been prescribed."
— **Resuscitation Council (UK)**

Not Permitted

- Using **Patient B's prescribed adrenaline auto-injector** to treat **Patient A**, even in an emergency.

Example Scenario

- Patient A develops anaphylaxis during dental treatment.
- Patient B (in the waiting room) has a prescribed adrenaline auto-injector.

Unlawful: Using Patient B's auto-injector on Patient A
Lawful:

- Using the **practice's emergency adrenaline auto-injector**, or
- Drawing up and administering **IM adrenaline from a practice-held ampoule**

INDEX

GLOSSARY

(Plain-English definitions for learners and CPD assessment)

ABCDE / DRS ABC
A structured clinical assessment used to identify and treat life-threatening problems in order: Danger, Response, Airway, Breathing, Circulation (± Disability, Exposure).

AED (Automated External Defibrillator)
A portable device that analyses heart rhythm and delivers a shock if a shockable cardiac arrest rhythm is detected.

Anaphylaxis
A severe, rapid-onset, life-threatening allergic reaction causing airway, breathing, and/or circulation compromise.

Anaphylactic shock
The most severe form of anaphylaxis, characterised by persistent hypotension and circulatory failure.

Angina
Chest discomfort caused by reduced blood flow to the heart muscle; may be stable or unstable.

Asystole
A non-shockable cardiac arrest rhythm with no electrical activity ("flatline").

Bag-Valve-Mask (BVM)
A handheld device used to deliver positive-pressure ventilation with oxygen.

Basic Life Support (BLS)
Immediate life-saving care for cardiac arrest, including CPR and defibrillation, until advanced care arrives.

Cardiac Arrest
The sudden cessation of effective heart function, leading to unconsciousness and absence of normal breathing.

Chain of Survival
A sequence of actions that maximise survival from cardiac arrest: early recognition, early CPR, early defibrillation, advanced care, and recovery.

Chest Compressions
Manual compressions of the chest to circulate blood during cardiac arrest.

Consent
A patient's voluntary and informed agreement to receive care or treatment.

Defibrillation
Delivery of an electrical shock to terminate a shockable cardiac arrest rhythm and allow normal rhythm to resume.

DNACPR
A clinical decision indicating that CPR should not be attempted if cardiac arrest occurs.

Hypoxia
Insufficient oxygen supply to tissues.

Oropharyngeal Airway (OPA)
A rigid airway adjunct used to prevent the tongue from obstructing the airway in an unconscious patient.

PEA (Pulseless Electrical Activity)
A non-shockable cardiac arrest rhythm where electrical activity is present, but no pulse is detectable.

Pulse Oximeter
A non-invasive device that measures oxygen saturation and pulse rate.

Rescue Breaths
Ventilations delivered during CPR to provide oxygen.

SBAR
A structured communication tool: Situation, Background, Assessment, Recommendation.

Shockable Rhythms
Cardiac arrest rhythms (VF and pulseless VT) that can be treated with defibrillation.

SpO₂
Peripheral oxygen saturation measured by pulse oximetry.

Ventricular Fibrillation (VF)
A shockable cardiac arrest rhythm with chaotic ventricular electrical activity.

Ventricular Tachycardia (VT)
A rapid ventricular rhythm; pulseless VT is a shockable cardiac arrest rhythm.

Bibliography

CARDIAC ARREST

Acute Coronary syndrome

STEMI

(Vogel B, Claessen BE, Arnold SV, et al. ST-segment elevation myocardial infarction. *Nat Rev Dis Primers*. 2019;5 (1):39. doi:10.1038/s41572-019-0090-3)

"Immediate Life Support," Resuscitation Council UK. 5th Edition P17-

18, 2021

"ST segment elevation myocardial infarction, the most severe type of heart attack "by Richard .N. Fogoros MD "Cardiac Biomarkers,
Cardiac enzymes, and heart disease" by Richard N Fogoros, dec 10,

2021

NICE-clinical guidelines 50 Acutely ill adults in hospital London, National Institute for health and clinical Excellence 2007 https://www.nice.org.uk/guidance/cg50

National institute for health and care excellence. Clinical guidelines 167 Myocardial infarction with ST-segment elevation . NICE 2013 www.nice.org.uk/guidance

Nolan JP, J, Smith GB et al Incidence and outcome of in hospital Cardiac arrest in the United Kingdom National Cardiac arrest audit.

Resuscitation 2014, 85:98987-92

Resuscitation council guidelines for safer handling during resuscitation in healthcare settings July 2015 http://www.resus.org.uk/library/publications/publication-guidance-saferhandling

AIRWAY MANAGEMENT

Airway management in cardiopulmonary resuscitation BY Jasmeet

Soar and Jerry P. Nolan CURRENT OPINION

DNAR

Do not attempt cardiopulmonary resuscitation (DNACPR) decisions -

NHS (www.nhs.uk)

ADRT (Advanced decision to refuse treatment)

Advance decision to refuse treatment - Macmillan Cancer Support

CARDIOPULMONARY RESUSCITATION (CPR)

UK resuscitation Council guidelines 2021

CHOKING

About 380 people die from choking every year and most of the deaths are those within the age of 65 years and over

ONS, 2017

Office for National Statistics, 2017. Deaths Registered in England and Wales.

Available at:
https://www.ons.gov.uk/peoplepopulationandcommunity/
birthsdeathsandmarriages/deaths/datasets/deathsregisteredineng
land

Causes, Prevention, and Treatment of Choking (verywellhealth.com)

Walls, 2012

Walls RM and Murphy MF (eds), 2012. Manual of Emergency Airway

Management. 4th ed. Philadelphia: Wolters Kluwer/Lippincott Williams & Wilkins Health.

What should I do if someone is choking? - NHS (www.nhs.uk)

www.ingramcontent.com/pod-product-compliance
Lightning Source LLC
Chambersburg PA
CBHW051246020426
42333CB00025B/3073